SPEAK the
LANGUAGE of
HEALING

SPEAK the LANGUAGE of HEALING

Living with Breast Cancer without Going to War

SUSAN KUNER, ED.D.

CAROL MATZKIN ORSBORN, M.T.S.

LINDA QUIGLEY, M.A.

KAREN LEIGH STROUP, M.DIV., PH.D.

Preface by Dr. Joycelyn Elders

Foreword by Jean Shinoda Bolen, M.D.

CONARI PRESS

First published in 1993 by Conari Press, an imprint of Red Wheel/Weiser LLC, with offices at 368 Congress Street, Fourth Floor, Boston, Massachusetts 02210.

ISBN: 1-57324-168-7

Cover photography: Teresa Vargo, Mill Valley, CA
Cover and Interior Design: Suzanne Albertson
Cover Art Direction: Ame Beanland

Library of Congress Cataloging-in-Publication Data

Speak the language of healing : living with breast cancer without going to war /
    Susan Kuner . . . [et al.]: forward by Jean Shinoda Bolen, M.D. :
    preface by Dr. Joycelyn Elders.
        p. cm.
    Includes index
    ISBN 1-57324-168-7
        1. Breast—Cancer—Psychological aspects. 2. Breast—Cancer—
    Religious aspects. 3. Mental healing. 4. Catastrophic illness. 5. Medicine,
    Psychosomatic. Metaphor.
    RC280.B8S588   1999
    362.1'9399449'0019—dc21   99-16073
                                                          CIP

Printed in the United States of America on recycled paper.

09 08 07 06 05   DR   10 9 8 7 6 5 4 3 2

To our fellow initiates, whose spiritual paths have led them into strange, new lands:

May this book serve as a companion and friend to you along the way.

SPEAK the LANGUAGE of HEALING

Preface

Dr. Joycelyn Elders,
former Surgeon General of the United States

THE DICTIONARY DEFINES *WAR* AS "any act or state of hostility; enmity; or conflict," and *to wage war* is "to be in any state of active opposition." These four women—Susan Kuner, Carol Matzkin Orsborn, Linda Quigley, and Karen Leigh Stroup—faced the terrifying diagnosis of breast cancer and courageously refused to go to war against their own bodies. For them, the disease was not an enemy to be vanquished but a part of themselves to explore, understand, and accept. As they confronted a medical establishment that spoke about the "war on cancer," with winners and losers, victims and survivors, they discovered that instead of adopting a vocabulary of conflict and competition, they could develop a new language with which to describe their experience— a language they hope will begin to shift the way we view life-threatening illness.

We need to be aggressive in our approach to diseases such as breast cancer, which threatens the life of one in every eight women in America. But an aggressive approach in terms of allocating resources, funding research, improving education, and extending treatment does not mean going to war. For some, the military metaphors may prove helpful, but particularly for women, there has to be room for relationship and integration, room to embrace life in all its parts, and room in which to heal. We must learn to refrain from speaking in polarities: the either/ors that reduce us to winners or losers, guilty or innocent, and that strip life of its mysteries and richness.

I applaud these four brave women for forging a new path when so much was at stake. They have four very different stories to tell, but the four stories tell one truth: Disease is not the target, death is not the enemy, and life is for celebrating, in all its brilliant, surprising, and complex fragments.

Foreword

Jean Shinoda Bolen, M.D.
author of *Close to the Bone*

THIS BOOK IS AN HONEST AND HEARTFELT REPORT from four women who were diagnosed and treated for breast cancer. Friendship, affinity, and synchronicity brought them together and gave birth to this book. The four women draw sustenance from four different spiritual traditions; and among them, the four women have Stage I, II, III, and IV cancers.

These four writers found they were kindred souls who did not wish to live on a battlefield, define themselves as survivors, or become part of a cancer culture. They found that heroic stories could be depressing, that being in control was neither possible nor desirable, and that they did not want to be drafted into the war against cancer. If anything, each found that cancer was a ticket to a deeper place on her spiritual, individual, human journey. Rather than a war model, theirs is a learning and healing model, for which a new vocabulary or language was needed for the cancer experience that they advocate in this book.

As those that investigate remissions know, in the treatment of cancer of the breast, something works for someone, and nothing works for everyone. I think that this principle applies to psychological attitudes as well. One's attitude toward having cancer does matter, but what works for one woman doesn't work for every woman. Sometimes being in the trenches and front lines is an apt description for what it feels like to have cancer, and having a fighting spirit is the right metaphor. Sometimes an inner warrior does need to be called forth. Some women do join the war against cancer and its causes once they are in remission, and many others do see themselves, in a positive light, as survivors. What is appropriate for some women does not apply to all. In their individual reactions, each of these four authors rejected battlefield metaphors as not true for them, which I know is also the case for many other women who will find themselves in good company as they read this book.

Each of the four authors tells her own story, beginning with the impact of the diagnosis and what happened next—as an inner and outer narrative. Each has her own experience to tell about the circumstances, what was done, and how others reacted, but much more significant and important to the reader is the recounting of what each woman felt and thought, what each rejected and accepted, questioned and learned throughout this ordeal.

From Impact, to Chaos, to Choices, to Community, to Spirit—each woman tells her version of the story in these stages. Without the vocabulary of myth, which I used in *Close to the Bone: Life-Threatening Illness and the Search for Meaning* to describe cancer as a descent of the soul into the underworld and an initiation, these women tell their stories from a spiritual perspective. For we are spiritual beings on a human path, rather than human beings who may or may not be on a spiritual path. Cancer may allow us or compel us to acknowledge what we know in our bones to be true, may turn us inward, and make our relationship with God a crucial issue. Cancer raises questions about guilt and suffering, about meaning and faith, about contradictions and mystery, and thus about God.

By telling us what was so for them, they contribute to a consciousness-raising perspective for others. For example, "The diagnosis of breast cancer is like a Rorschach test. Everybody ascribes the cause to their worst fear." Or, on having to make medical choices: "The truth is, the questions that we are really being asked to answer are things like: How badly do I want to live? How important is physical beauty to me? How strong is my faith? My willingness to endure pain? What's my life about?" Or, "No one knows how to have cancer." Or, one simple important lesson: "The dishes can wait."

I was told that cancer was once called "the wisdom disease." I think it still is. Learning you have a disease that could kill you puts life in a spiritual perspective, makes you think about what really matters and who really matters. As these four women found, having cancer provides lessons in perspective. Each of us gets our share and kind of suffering as an inevitable part of being human: what happens in us as a result makes all the difference to the psyche. Cancer makes us aware of death and the preciousness of life, usually allows time to reflect about what is important and what is trivial, and provides opportunities for healing and learning. Cancer can be a wisdom disease because it allows time to make choices, to forgive and set straight, to face what we fear, and find unexpected gifts, strengths, vulnerabilities, and joys. This is what these authors found separately, and then in reading each other's stories, were moved to tears with a realization of the paradox: We are alone here, and yet at a profound level, we are not alone.

HOW THIS BOOK
CAME TO BE

Carol Matzkin Orsborn

WHEN I WAS FIRST DIAGNOSED WITH BREAST CANCER, well-meaning friends gave me a number of books that alternately encouraged me to "run the race for my life," "wage war against the enemy," and achieve the ultimate goal: to be a "survivor." Not only did I have to deal with all the emotions anyone would feel when facing her mortality, but I was asked to assume a competitive, warlike value system that was opposite to my own innate sense of how life was meant to be lived. Of course I wanted to live—but not as a "survivor," not as someone who would let a reactive relationship to a disease define her entire existence.

Happily, I was blessed with inspirational role models: three remarkable women who were on the journey through breast cancer a few steps ahead of me and who had independently arrived at similar conclusions. Miraculously, all of them came to me at a critical moment, bringing with them their own wisdom and experience. As I went through the stages of diagnosis, treatment, and recovery, I often called on their friendship as well as their expertise.

The first woman was Dr. Susan Kuner, who was already my best friend in Nashville. In fact, it was the diagnosis of Susan's breast cancer that alerted me to my own developing situation—quite possibly saving my life. As I sat at the foot of her bed on and off during the early months of her illness—and before I knew I, too, had a problem—I watched in awe as Susan entered her new territory with all the aplomb of a spiritual pioneer. Her remarkable journey was a major influence on the upbeat philosophy underlying the book I was writing at the time: *The Art of Resilience: One Hundred Paths to Wisdom and Strength in an Uncertain World.* Ironically, by the time that book was published, it was Susan's turn to sit with me. Not only did I have a mastectomy, but my more serious diagnosis called for months of chemotherapy treatment she had not needed.

In the midst of treatment, doing what I could to promote my book while dealing with the physical effects of chemo, including the loss of my hair, Linda Quigley, a feature writer for the *Tennessean,* came to the house to interview me for the paper. I must have been the only person in Nashville who didn't know that Linda had also had breast cancer and undergone chemotherapy. In fact, she had written about her experiences the previous year in the daily paper, receiving a top award for her writing. As the interview proceeded, it soon became obvious that we not only had breast cancer in common, but an excitement about the spiritual dimensions the disease was opening up for us.

At the time I was promoting my book, I was also in the midst of completing the two final courses of my Master of Theological Studies degree at Vanderbilt University's Divinity School. Everyone who heard about my situation at school had the same response: You've got to talk to Karen Stroup. Karen had been diagnosed with breast cancer while pursuing her doctorate in religion several years before me. But somehow I didn't get around to it—and then during an unplanned moment in the chemotherapy treatment room, I finally met the Reverend Doctor Karen Leigh Stroup—yet another serendipitously life-changing encounter. Karen, who I am proud to say is now my friend, reached out to me at a particularly scary moment to teach me how to hope against the odds. Not only do we now have a serious theological education from Vanderbilt University in common, but an unbounded belief in miracles, as well.

When I finally finished chemotherapy, just one year ago, I gave myself permission to put my experiences behind me and return to the book topics that I had begun before diagnosis, one about my experiences at divinity school and another about spirituality at work. Frankly, I didn't want to dwell on the details of my illness—not even the inspirational ones. Unfortunately, my own return to everyday life was too often interrupted by phone calls from women newly entering the world of breast cancer and other serious illnesses. Could I offer them any advice? I did what I could. But one thought kept coming back to me: They needed not only to hear from me, but from my friends, as well. The urgency of my mission picked up tempo as I increasingly encountered the "cancer culture": a world in which people who die are "losers," and the "winners" are those who emerge from illness unchanged. I knew that this unhealthy attitude was useful in that it heightened emotions around our illness in order to raise funds for research more effectively, but it came at the expense of our spirits. As a seasoned author of spiritual books, I had long ago given up the idea of being a master of the universe. I'd learned to stop thinking of my inner world and outer challenges as enemies to be conquered, and learned to recognize the potential for true greatness in acceptance and compassion for myself and for others, regardless of the obstacles I faced. To create the optimum environment for my healing—body, mind, and spirit—what I most needed was not a mighty sword but rather a mighty heart: a heart that could hope, love, and remain faithful in the shadow of mysteries that were beyond my comprehension. This was my prayer: to grow my connection to God through my deepening humility.

One day, after leaving a fund-raiser exhorting us to lead the charge in the war against cancer, I decided to make four phone calls, one to each of my friends, and a fourth to agent Linda Roghaar. How about writing a book about cancer that challenged the war mentality and that supported readers to create a new kind of relationship to their disease— a spiritual relationship that would truly create the environment in which the deepest healing possible could take place? This healing, I knew, could take place regardless of the outcome. Because these three women were my teachers as well as friends, I knew they would understand.

Joyously, there were four "Yes's" to the idea for this book. Soon thereafter, there was a fifth "Yes," from Conari Press, who recognized and supported the radical nature of what we were trying to do. Together, we agreed on nine key questions we wanted to address. We realized that the questions followed an order. We recognized common and identifiable issues and stages. We grouped our questions into five broad topics or stages, the psychological and spiritual landmarks those who face life-threatening disease routinely encounter.

Working independently after that first meeting, each of us answered the questions from our individual spiritual perspective, derived from personal experience. Ensuring our own fresh voices and perspectives— while continuing to grow our friendships on a personal level—we eagerly anticipated the time in the not-too-distant future when we would come together again to share our answers. You'll see that while we arrive at similar places, we often get there via very different routes. We hope that by showing you our most intimate relationships to cancer, we can help you find your own path through illness as spiritual initiation rather than war.

When I invited my three fellow writers to join this project, I knew that this mission—the desire to chart a new pathway through illness— was something we had in common. What I hadn't stopped to realize is that we had as many differences between us as we had similarities. Among the four of us, we represented four (or more) different spiritual traditions and four different stages of breast cancer: Stages I, II, III, and IV. Susan, with Stage I cancer, studied for more than twenty-five years with a Sufi teacher, Pir Vilayat Khan. Linda, with Stage III, grew her spirituality within the twelve-step programs. Karen, Stage IV, is Christian and a minister of a church. I am Jewish, a theologian, and a student of Eastern philosophy. My cancer is Stage II.

We also represent a diversity of living arrangements and choices, with and without children, husbands, or partners.

What we share, however, is the discovery that even something as frightening as breast cancer can be incorporated into a full and joyful life. As you read this book, I believe you will become attuned to hearing not only in our voices but, in many voices, the growing grassroots aware-ness of the spiritual dimensions of serious illness. Wherever you are in your journey through life, I invite you to join our quiet revolution.

HOW TO HAVE CANCER
WITHOUT GOING TO WAR

THE WOMEN OF THE BABY BOOM GENERATION have changed every institution we've touched. We've changed the way women work, parent, relate to men and to each other, how we dress—even down to our undergarments. We are, after all, the same generation that burned our bras in the 1960s. We have come to understand hot flashes as power surges and view aging as the new frontier in which we redefine midlife and beyond.

Now, sadly, we have a new task: transforming the world of breast cancer and other serious illnesses, with their rampant macho terminology of warfare and survival, winning and losing. This quiet revolution is largely a spiritual movement, already well underway, as individual women experience their own brushes with mortality not as tests of survivorship but as initiations into the deeper mysteries of life. For a growing number of us, life-threatening illness carries with it spiritual dimensions and meanings that the current crop of advice books in the field does not even come close to touching.

Women are giving voice to a new way of viewing disease. We want to describe the experience of cancer in a different language. There is a spiritual pathway through cancer, a new language to express ourselves and to speak with others.

Of course we want the scientific facts, the medical research, the latest technology—not to mention the inspirational stories of women who beat the odds. But we want something more. Regardless of the outcome of our illness, we want a quality of life that reflects our deepest values.

The feminine values of coexistence instead of separation, integration instead of banishment, and relationship instead of opposition clash with our experiences of the health care system. The landscape is jarring. With full memories of our generation's marches for peace, we find that our culture is waging a "war" on cancer. People with cancer are either "victims" or "survivors." When a women dies, her obituary says, "She lost her battle with cancer." Our doctors and friends encourage us to be upbeat and to maintain a "fighting spirit." Get a cancer diagnosis, and you will find yourself at war.

> Imagine that our nation is at war. The war drags on for years, and the years turn into decades. The government announces that, in the last year alone, the war cost over half a million American lives—hundreds of thousands more deaths than World War II. That's actually what has happened in the war on cancer, declared 25 years ago by President Nixon.

This quote is from publicity for "The March," a grassroots movement that demonstrated against the enemy—cancer—hoping government would increase funding for research. That's a noble cause, but listen further to the language:

> It will be the biggest Hallelujah Chorus in history. A grand and glorious noise. The echo of a million voices, speaking as one. It is called The March. The last mile in the journey that will conquer cancer. The final proof that the irresistible force of human spirit can defeat the immoveable object of disease.

The honorary chairperson of The March was General Norman Schwarzkopf, the military leader of Desert Storm. When we heard him talk on television about The March, he sounded much like he did when he was planning an attack on the Persian Gulf.

The world of life-threatening disease is frequently described as a battle. Our language comes from our culture, and the choices are few. Battle language offers strength and encouragement when navigating the strange and frightening process of life-threatening disease. The battle language is not wrong. No way of coping with cancer is wrong. Some research even indicates that a fighting spirit may prolong survival.

Each person must find her own way, digging for footholds in a steep, craggy terrain. But what about those of us who do not see life as a battle? Winning words and battle language do not describe our experiences or attitudes. Carol tells how she found herself on the battlefield at a cancer fund-raiser.

> As I approached the end of chemotherapy, I received an invitation to attend my first cancer fund-raiser. I was excited by the promise of being in a room with so many other women who had gone through the cancer experience. I thought it would be healing for me. I invited Susan to come along. When she hesitated, I was astonished.
>
> Then I found out why. A step ahead of me, Susan had already dipped her toe in the cancer culture. She tried to warn me, but I plunged right in.
>
> The women at my table were great—everything I had hoped for. I would have loved to have had more time to talk with them. But too soon our attention was called to the front of the room. Over a box lunch, the talk from the podium was not about healing, but about warfare. The keynote address was delivered by an energetic TV actress, who bounded about the stage, demonstrating how she had used the strength of her will to kick cancer's butt. A self-avowed superwoman, cancer was no match for her. Through positive thinking, she had accomplished what lesser mortals sometimes failed to do: rid herself of all signs of the disease.
>
> She was followed by a tough-as-nails public official, a woman in her sixties who was receiving an honor for her legislative work in support of the fight against cancer. She used the occasion to brag about her victory over cancer: making it to work every single day of her treatment. She had emerged from the battle virtually unchanged. With reconstructive surgery, she had the breasts of a twenty-year-old.

Although none of us viewed breast cancer as war, it was all too easy to find ourselves drafted.

Sports have many similarities with war, one being that we are either winners or losers. Susan tells this story:

> The event was a cancer fund-raiser, one of thousands like it in cities and towns around the country. So many people had lost loved ones. This was their way of giving back, of raising needed dollars for research, treatment, prevention, and for a cure.
>
> The theme was a race. At the track of a suburban school, people arrived with tents, coolers, and lawn chairs. The walkers and runners were to circle the track night and day. Participants had solicited donations for their journeys.
>
> This was my first outing at a public cancer event. Emerging from the almost full-time job of being a cancer patient, I wanted to join the movement.
>
> The track looked like a carnival. At the tent with a sign for our hospital, I spotted Carol and her family.
>
> The crowd was upbeat. But for Carol and me, this gaiety was weird and confusing. We clung to each other. Carol was still in chemotherapy. Her port, the tube allowing easy entry for the chemotherapy concoctions, was sutured into her chest, hidden beneath her blouse. She wore a floppy hat on her bald head. My treatment had ended months earlier.
>
> At the sponsor's tent, "survivors" signed in. The survivors, bearing balloons and sashes, were invited to walk the initial lap.
>
> We lined up on the track and began to walk. A friend from graduate school was beside me. He has cancer? I hadn't known. He had been diagnosed with Stage IV lymphoma, a cancer of the lymphatic system. I recalled my cancer statistics, which since my diagnosis I had studied as if for cate-

chism. The tables say he has a small chance of survival. In cancer terms, survival means living for five years. There on the track, we made a date for lunch.

We had no time to talk further because a roar erupted from the crowd. People were shouting and applauding madly. "Why on earth are they clapping for us?" I thought. "Because we have cancer and are still alive? In the past, when people applauded, it was because of something we had accomplished. This was not our choice." I didn't get it. But we had completed one lap. We crossed the finish line. The applause was for our metaphoric accomplishment.

Carol and I had an important talk that evening. Her surgery was behind her. Well, almost. In addition to the port, a second plastic tube with a bulb on the end snaked out of her mastectomy incision to drain the wound of liquids. The plumbing aspect of cancer is hidden from the public. The ones who are treated know it well. It is bizarre and uncomfortable, but quite tolerable and even welcome on the scale of dreadful possibilities. The surgical drain speeds healing. The port replaces needle sticks.

Carol was despondent. She was ready to get back into the activities of her life. Her experimental chemotherapy treatments would last for several more months, but had become manageable. Two days of feeling dead, a few days of transition, and by the end of the week, feeling more or less like herself. A determined, energetic woman of many accomplishments, why did she feel so exhausted and unsure? "What's wrong with me?" she had been asking. At this stage she had pictured herself well on the road to recovery.

Healing takes time. Time to recover physically from the treatment, the shock of surgery, and the sheer toxicity of the chemotherapy agents. It takes time for the body to find its equilibrium again. It takes time to learn to live with cancer as a chronic disease. It takes time to get used to the uncertainty of a disease where great advances have been made, but the cause remains unknown. It takes time to reorient the body, mind, and spirit to a life profoundly changed.

I told her about the rule of thumb I had developed. Physically, with my excellent prognosis and nearly a year out from my treatment, I should have been back to my old self. Instead, I was dealing with sudden waves of sadness and loss. My rule of thumb was this:

If I cry at the office, I stay. If I sob, I go home.

Carol was surprised. She was ready for this to be over. Determined, savvy, spiritual, supported by family and friends, insured, receiving excellent medical treatment, she seemed to have everything going for her. Like the race, why couldn't she just use her will to cross the finish line? She was relieved to hear that even with the acute treatment over, it was not clear sailing. She saw that uncertainty could be just as much a part of healing as a positive attitude.

The four of us wrote this book to suggest that there are ways one can have cancer without going to war. As you will see in our stories, we are women for whom the war metaphor just didn't work. Yet, when we told the medical establishment that "winning the battle" in no way described our experiences, many assumed we had a death wish. Wrong. We had a life wish, a wish to integrate our experiences with cancer. Cancer was not an enemy to be vanquished, but a part of ourselves. Thank goodness we found each other. We know there are many more like us.

We see why the battle metaphor for cancer persists. The tumor is the enemy. With our doctors, we make a battle plan. Surgery. Chemotherapy. Radiation. The tumor recedes. With diagnostic tests and physical exams, we scan the horizon. A new tumor may appear. Another treatment. Another skirmish. And so it goes. The good news is that because of research, treatments are improving and a person can live this way for a long time.

But the danger of this battle metaphor is that the spread of disease may become the measure of the fight. We cry for the harm it does to those who feel they did not fight hard enough, who fear that death means, "I lose." Many people suffer unnecessary anguish because of this belief.

More sensitivity is being developed about the harm of the battle image. For example, the cancer support organization Gilda's Club asks all presenters to refrain from dwelling on the fighting spirit, eliminating words like *struggle* and *battle*. The path of spirit is not the path of competition and war. The path of spirit finds a way to unify jagged fragments, to make a patchwork quilt out of what might have been discarded or despised.

This is the feminine way of being in the world. In the *Odyssey*, while Odysseus was at war, Penelope stayed home weaving. For many centuries, it has been Odysseus who has been the more highly regarded, the adventurer in foreign lands, the conquering hero. Now, the perspective is shifting to the feminine in many aspects of our culture.

In various fields we are learning that the world is an interdependent place, a globe that has put people in such close contact that the only hope is cooperation and coexistence. For instance, Celeste White writes in an article about microbes in the Institute of Noetic Sciences newsletter that, "instead of talking about war, we should be asking how we can interact successfully with infectious microorganisms." That enemy is not outside us, but is part of us. In the awakening of consciousness, we are no longer missionaries to other lands. To change the world, we must start with ourselves.

The role model for women and men is no longer Odysseus the Hero, but Penelope the Weaver. Suddenly we see that the work of Penelope, staying right where she is, is much more important for our time. We must study how things fit together, and how to work with systems instead of their parts. There is no enemy and no one to blame.

We want to change more than the words we use to talk about cancer. Words correspond to consciousness, to an awakening in a world that is much more than it seems. Perhaps even more distressing than her illness to a woman who has been diagnosed is the fact that this wider consciousness is often missing from the medical system and from our communities.

When each of the four of us was diagnosed with breast cancer, many friends tried to be helpful. We are grateful for their consideration, support, and concern. We received many self-help books about fighting disease. Some were encouraging. Most felt preachy and annoying. They were often either patronizingly sunny or summonses to battle. They did not leave room for the infinite number of tiny steps through the maze of emotions that come with a life-threatening illness. The authors of those books wanted us to banish demons that we had not yet gotten to know. Susan tells the story of one of these tiny steps in the maze:

> One month after my diagnosis, I sat in my usual decision-making posture: half dressed, perched on the edge of the examining table. My surgeon was telling me that the news was not good. I had been adamant about saving my breast, and responding to my wishes, he had performed a lumpectomy. He found a second tumor in the tissue surrounding the first. This confirmed his initial diagnosis. Multi-focal breast disease. Treatment of choice: mastectomy.
>
> I finally agreed. I had tried so hard to save my breast. I was worn down and exhausted.
>
> "Before we go into surgery," he said, "I need to know if you want breast reconstruction."
>
> I could not deal with one more question. I burst into tears. "I don't know how to have cancer," I sobbed.
>
> He touched me gently on the shoulder. "No one knows how to have cancer."

We would never claim, nor would we want to, that we know how to have cancer. Yet after reading each other's accounts, we know much more. Through our diagnoses, treatments, research, and questions, we were convinced that a deeper level of information was available somehow, somewhere. The scientific research was useful but inconclusive. The heroic tales of overcoming illness were depressing. We needed real, honest, considered, balanced, spiritual accounts of experience. We needed multiple perspectives. We needed hope that was grounded in reality. We needed a new description of the critical pathway through disease and a new language with which to talk about it.

This book is by four women who have cancer and who do not wish to live on a battlefield. We have times when we fight, other times when we surrender, but we are not at war. We are at peace. At least we try to be, in the moments when the turmoil dies down or when clarity shines. We want to go out on the edge, learn the most we can, from the widest range of emotions. We are not afraid to cry in anguish, rant in frustration, and laugh uproariously. Rather than ask, "Why me?" we say, "Come what may."

We wish we could say that none of you will have to take this path of breast cancer, that we were the only four who would have to travel this journey. But we know some of you will join us, or will care for someone who does. So until we understand the cause of this disease and can find a way to prevent it, we present a framework for the path of illness.

This critical pathway is divided into five broad steps, the psychological and spiritual landmarks of a disease that can mean death. Although one would never choose illness, it can serve as a catalyst for understanding. With spiritual preparation or with grace, illness can open up a profound realization about the sacredness of life. In this sense, some would call cancer a gift; however, we've come to see that the gift is what we bring to the experience, not what it brings to us. We need new words and concepts to describe the next frontiers of care and understanding.

HOW TO SPEAK THE LANGUAGE OF HEALING

Instead of saying	Say
I am a victim of breast cancer.	I was diagnosed with breast cancer on...
I am a survivor.	I am a cancer initiate. I am living with a breast cancer diagnosis. It has been six years since my initial diagnosis.
I am fighting breast cancer.	I am in treatment for breast cancer.
I beat cancer.	I was initiated by cancer.
She lost her battle with breast cancer.	Breast cancer was the cause of her death.
The War on Cancer.	Advances in breast cancer research and treatment.
Chemotherapy is poison.	Chemotherapy is medicine.
How are you?	It's good to see you.
I am cured of cancer.	I am doing well.
Anything about God such as, "God must love you very much."	I will keep you in my thoughts; I will keep you in my prayers.
You'll be fine.	I hope it goes well for you.
Did they get it all?	I hope it went well.
Is there anything I can do?	Be specific in your offers: can I get your groceries, pick up your kids...

A PATHWAY TO SPIRIT:
THE FIVE STAGES
OF TRANFORMATION

THIS PATH OF DEALING WITH A LIFE-THREATENING ILLNESS is full of surprises and uneven terrain. The landscape can change abruptly. These stages may go in order or loop back on themselves. They follow the alchemical cycle that is the essential cycle of nature. In Latin these stages are called "dissolve" and "coagule." They mean falling apart and coming together. The Stage of Impact, and The Stage of Chaos, are on the falling-apart side of the cycle. The Stage of Choices is a difficult and critical turning point. The Stage of Community, and The Stage of Spirit, are the coming-together part of the cycle, the stages of healing. We describe these stages in four parts: the triggering events, the questions you may ask yourself, the underlying issues, and what others can do. This last is especially important. Often people are at a loss for what to do or say to a person with cancer. Part of this depends on where the person with cancer is on the path. We offer some suggestions for each of the stages.

A Pathway to Spirit: The Five Stages of Transformation

	Questions	Events	Inner Thoughts	Others' Support
Impact	Did I create this?	Cancer diagnosis.	No one knows the cause of cancer. No one can be prepared.	Hold you, hug you, be with you, let you cry.
Chaos	Does death mean I lose? Will God help or am I on my own? Does God get to vote?	Shock of diagnosis. Telling others.	Facing death. Relationship with a power greater than ourselves.	Facing death is a life wish, not a death wish. Resist the urge to say, "Everything will be all right," or that God gave you this.
Choices	Is treatment war or initiation? Do I hold on or do I let go? Do I trust the medical establish-ment or put my faith in alterna-tive and spiritual healing?	Learning about treatment choices. Deciding what to do. Having treatment. Following your chosen path.	Learning to trust. There are many alternatives. There is no one "right" way. Spirit includes science and vice versa.	Support your treatment choices. Enter your view of cancer and speak from it.
Community	From whom must I learn to receive? From whom must I learn to protect myself?	Treatment ending. Recovering from treatment. Living without the assurance of active treatment. Putting a life back together.	Trust your intuition. Accept that some people's influence can be harmful. Ask for what you need. Seek support in whatever form works for you.	Realize that it is not over for you. Stay with you through the ups and downs.
Spirit	How can I find peace of mind when I'm living my life over the edge? What have I learned?	Looking back. Looking forward.	Digesting the experience. Whatever happens in life IS your spiritual path. Gently guiding others through this terrain.	Learn from you.

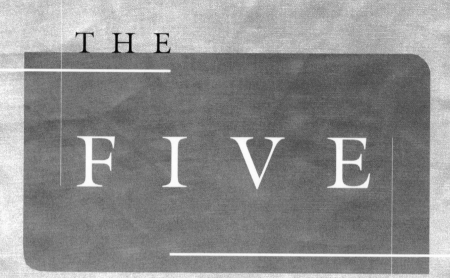

THE FIVE

STAGES OF
TRANSFORMATION

Impact

THIS STAGE HAS A CLEAR MARKER: the dreaded words, "You have cancer." One of the first questions that may come to your mind is, "Did I create this?" This is a stage of shock and disbelief. No matter what comes next, nothing will ever be the same.

No one knows the cause of cancer, and no one can be prepared for it. However, at this stage, we forget those things at first. We have heard so much about medical advances; where are they when we need them? We are so used to being in control. That control is gone.

> *What lies behind us and what lies before us*
> *are small matters, compared to*
> *what lies within us.*
> —RALPH WALDO EMERSON

When the diagnosis of breast cancer is delivered—and it will be for one out of eight American women—one of the most painful issues we encounter is how and what we contributed to the development of the disease.

The four of us who are additions to the statistics would say "No" if we were asked if we caused our breast cancer. Some aspects of our lifestyles might have impacted it, might have brought it sooner rather than later, but we are not responsible for it.

It *is* our responsibility to embrace cancer and its impact on our bodies and our psyches—anger, shock, grief, loss, and fear, as well as courage, self-love, acceptance, and, eventually, humor and joy. It is there that we find maps for the journey, light for the darkness, and nourishment for the soul.

For many of us, cancer is our ticket to a spiritual journey that will find us, like the Ancient Mariner, blessing it unaware. Granted, it isn't the trip we'd planned—no, sorry, we're all out of tickets to Disneyland—but it's one that ultimately can be as rewarding as it is painful, as enriching as it is debilitating.

No, you did not cause it, your sister did not cause it, your mother did not cause it. It arrived unbidden, even though there were perhaps hints along the way, and now it is yours to shape into a piece of your heart and soul. And that is what you, with the spiritual tools of your understanding, can be responsible for causing and can take the credit for creating.

Did I Create This?

Carol

In the Jewish Scriptures, it is written that every forty-ninth year there is to be a Jubilee Year. In the Jubilee Year, all debts are forgiven and everyone is given a fresh start. As I approached my forty-ninth birthday, I knew that something big was going to happen that was going to change my life forever. I never imagined that the vehicle would be breast cancer. While my forty-ninth year was not always as joyful as I'd imagined a Jubilee Year to be, neither was it always painful. Ironically, through the emotional and spiritual processes that accompanied my year of diagnosis, treatment, and recovery, I now realize that I got everything a Jubilee Year promises and more: all my emotional debts have been forgiven. I am free in ways I never imagined possible for myself.

My Jubilee Year finds its spiritual roots in the day I went for my thirteenth routine mammogram. I remember that day as particularly rushed. Because I was so certain I was completely healthy, the annual ritual was a major inconvenience. I hurriedly filled in the form, telling them yet again that I had no known history of breast cancer in my family, I didn't smoke or drink, nor did I have any health problems. When the clerk behind the counter at the clinic couldn't locate my records, I was snippier than I would like to have been.

Imagine my shock when one week later, instead of a postcard from the clinic telling me I was fine, I got a phone call from the physician's office. There was something suspicious-looking in the mammogram that bore looking into further.

From that moment on, the history of my diagnosis of breast cancer was not a textbook situation, where indications were clearly given and treatment a logical outcome. In fact, through a comedy of errors, featuring misplaced mammograms, doctors on vacation, and mysteriously vanishing reports, the lump in my breast that I dismissed as part of my natural anatomy was witnessed by three respected physicians and radiologists who told me not to worry—and one who told me I should.

I chose to listen to the doctors who told me not to worry—to come back in a year as prescribed for a routine checkup. But four months after that controversial mammogram, my best friend Susan was diagnosed with breast cancer. I put off a return visit to my physician for another four months. Sure, I could have been more aggressive earlier. I could have paid attention to the one physician out of the pack who sounded the warning bell. But it is also true that I tend to overreact to things. I don't want to be the kind of person who lets fear run her. So I waited it out, hoping it was nothing.

It wasn't.

Little had I known that my rushed and rude behavior on the day of my thirteenth mammogram was to take on mythic proportions in my life. How many times did I find myself asking, "Could my breast cancer be punishment for my rudeness that day? Did I think I was so much better than every other woman that I was never going to get a serious illness? What shadowy flaw was there in my soul and psyche that would have made such a diagnosis possible?"

In our society, we so desperately want to feel in control of our lives.

Self-help books, pop psychologists, and spiritual workshops all deliver the same message: You can learn to call the shots of your destiny. You just have to be strong enough, positive enough, good enough, smart enough, spiritual enough, and you can get what you want. Even within the cancer culture, celebrity poster people deliver the message that they beat their cancer through the strength of their wills: "If you have the stuff it takes, you, too, will be a survivor and win the war against cancer." It's easy to applaud the indomitability of the human spirit. But there's a price for the applause. For if you can, could, and should be able to kick cancer—if you do have it within your means to control your destiny—then *why did you create your cancer in the first place?*

"Why did you create your cancer?" is a question that lies deep in one's own unconscious. It is also a question that, unfortunately, was asked by supportive family and friends and even well-meaning strangers who gently suggested that I look at the part I played in creating my cancer. A friend delivered her diatribe against modern kitchen appliances with such conviction that, to the dismay of my husband and children, I unplugged the microwave oven and hid it in the garage. The vegetarian at my door assured me that, unlike me, she would never become a breast cancer statistic—and that if I knew what was good for me, I would swear off meat today. It took several days for me to remember that Linda McCartney, a committed vegetarian, had died of breast cancer. When I mentioned it to my vegetarian friend, she had an explanation: "She didn't stop eating meat early enough."

And then there are the metaphysical explanations. When your family and friends tell you that you were sent this painful situation as a lesson, that it is your karma, a gift, or even punishment, they are trying to be helpful. By proposing that you bear responsibility for your cancer—not only for what you've done in this life but the last, as well—the assumption is that you can now do something to fix the situation. Think more positively, cleanse your spirit, and the universe will make the bad thing go away.

In the days after diagnosis, I sought out the one holistic physician in town to see how I might go about supplementing Western medicine. I knew I was afraid and desperate. But I was determined to use every resource within my means to fight this thing.

Despite the mixed reviews this man had received from my circle of friends, I found him attentive to my plight. We talked. He prescribed odd herbs and powders to supplement my diet. Then he turned the lights down and the soothing music up, massaging the tension out of my muscles. As I lay there, beginning to feel trust and hope for the first time since diagnosis, he whispered in my ear, "You do know, don't you, that cancer is nothing more than socially acceptable suicide. None of this will do any good unless you ask yourself: 'Do I want to live or do I want to die?'"

His words sent shock waves up and down my spine. Could it be that my diagnosis was actually the fulfillment of an unconsciously held death wish? For several days, I was so ashamed of the possibility, I moped about, keeping what the doctor said a secret. Then, at last, I confided in my husband Dan. Over and over again, Dan reassured me that my fears were not an indication of how much I wanted to die, but how much I wanted to live.

"But maybe I needed this cancer as a wake-up call or something," I whimpered.

"You can't wake somebody up who's not asleep, Carol," Dan said. "You are the kind of person who gets valuable lessons from all the things that happen to you—even this. But that doesn't mean that you *needed* this. From my perspective, what I see is someone who is bringing the same vital spirit to breast cancer that she brings to everything she does!"

Dan's calming words made sense to me. Of course, it is true that we can learn from the things that happen to us. Often, we can even come to recognize that something good has come out of a situation we would rather have avoided. But did I create this in order to perfect myself in some way? Did God pick me out specially either for punishment or gift? If you cannot speak of lessons and gifts before a starving child in Rwanda, or the innocent victim of a drive-by shooting in Los Angeles, then you should not unthinkingly apply this notion of personal responsibility to breast cancer, either.

At these times you must have the courage to confront the possibility that what happened to you or to others contains no inherently useful meaning whatsoever. Sometimes the only lesson to be gleaned is that life brings with it no guarantees. Things don't always make sense. They are not always deserved. In the end, all we can know for certain is the mystery. We must look elsewhere than the illusion of personal power to find meaning in the midst of suffering.

It has taken every bit of these past several years to accept in the deepest levels of my being that being rushed, arrogant, or rude—or any of my other sins, real or imagined—does not cause breast cancer. Nor did I have a subconscious death wish. The fact that I got the phone call instead of the postcard from the clinic this time does not indicate that I am any more cavalier or stressed than any of my less statistically challenged sisters. Did I create my breast cancer because I worried about finding the best college for my son? Did my nurse create her breast cancer because of her divorce?

The diagnosis of breast cancer is like a Rorschach test. Everybody ascribes the cause to their worst fear. This one was emotionally blocked; that one was too fat. But if each of our worst fears were truly the cause, there would be no woman walking around with both her breasts today. For who among us hasn't had something to mourn, a problem in an important relationship, a sexual indiscretion . . . a something! The truth is, medical science simply does not know why any one of us—let alone so many of us—are getting breast cancer. They have some data, some thoughts, and some suspicions. But trust me, none of it corroborates any of the personal pet theories I clobbered myself over the head with from time to time after my diagnosis.

The fact that so many of us are willing to ask and answer the question, "Why did I create this?" is an indication of how terrified we are of losing control. The alternative physician did me the greatest service when he voiced aloud my deepest fears. (But once was enough. I never went back!) Because of him, I came to realize that even my fears are an indication of the depth of the attachment I feel to living. Everything I've done in my life, and continue to do, has been for life, not death.

To refuse to take on the responsibility for creating my illness is to admit with deepest humility that I am human and so I am limited. I won't get through my life without butting up against problems. I won't even do breast cancer perfectly. But there is something I now know in the depth of my bones: I would rather live one day in the faith and love of my ordinary, vulnerable life than one hundred years burdened by the effort to maintain the illusion of control. Self-righteous vegetarians, past-life therapists, alternative caregivers, cancer poster people: Listen to me! It is not just about winning the battle. It's about choosing to live whatever life one has been blessed with to the fullest. This is our only real responsibility—not "Why did I create this disease?" but, "Will I create a meaningful life no matter what?"

Susan

I am sorting through breast cancer questions, like cleaning out an old drawer. I just celebrated the one-year anniversary of the end of my treatment. This was the year when I was initiated by cancer. A modern-day version of the Eleusian mysteries. Dressed in a hospital gown, or at my Breast Center in a pink bathrobe, I was dropped into the center of a dark labyrinth. The questions were my tasks.

It has been a year of crying—tears of loss and tears of gratitude. I never knew when they would come. And surprisingly, much laughter. Initiation is a step into the unknown. It is always accompanied by a test. The ones who make it through are profoundly changed.

Did I create this?

No. I never blamed myself. My grandmother got breast cancer at age thirty-five. The doctor told her to put salve on the lump. Within the year, she was dead. My mother was six years old, her brothers four and two. My mother was diagnosed at age sixty-five. She lived. When it was my turn, I thought it was part of my genetic inheritance over which I have no control. Hazel eyes. Size ten shoes. Breast cancer.

Having breast cancer is a public event. It seems as if I am always talking to people about cancer. Intimate talk with other women with this disease. Defensive talk with people who did not know what to say to me. The ones with that Oh-my-God-she's-going-to-die look in their eyes who said, "How are you?" but did not really want to know. I found women who blamed themselves. And people who blamed me. Everyone has a theory about cancer.

Variation #1: If Only. . .

I am on the phone with the friend of a friend. We have never met, but I often get calls like this. We are involuntary members of the same sorority, women with breast cancer. After twelve years, her cancer has returned. Since her initial diagnosis and treatment, she has made many changes in her life. She examined her priorities. She returned to graduate school. Her relationship with her husband has improved. She eats wholesome foods.

I tell her a little about myself. I too am in graduate school. When I get to the part about being a meditation teacher for the past twenty years, I hear her intake of breath.

"You meditate?" she asks.

"Yes," I answer. "Every day."

"And you still got cancer?"

"Yes."

She is shocked. And relieved. She had been meaning to learn to meditate. She never did get around to it. Now that her cancer has recurred, she could not shake the thought, "If I only had been meditating, my cancer would not have come back."

The language of blame and guilt runs like a subterranean current. We are not good enough, pure enough, vigilant enough, or smart enough to protect ourselves. We think "if only. . . ." Fill in the blank. If only we were more assertive. If only we ate better. If only we were thinner. If only we had not taken birth control pills. If only we meditated. At least I saved someone from that one. There is no end to the "if only's." Is there a way through this disease without regret?

Variation #2: Lead a Pure Life

I am standing by the clay spring-water dispenser at a reunion of old friends from the commune days. We ate tofu and macrobiotic food decades before the supermarkets had health food sections. One friend is still pure in his '60s ideals. He eats only vegetables, grains, nuts, and fruits. He has already sent me articles about how a vegetarian diet can prevent and cure cancer.

As I reach to fill the teapot from the sink, he asks why I do not use the spring water. I yell, "You think I got cancer because I drink tap water, don't you?" He is surprised by the intensity of my outburst. So am I. But not ashamed. Cancer has reduced my need to be polite.

I explain to him that his accusations are not helping me. That cancer has made my grip on life tenuous at best and that I feel fragile. I would much prefer to take a walk or have a hug than hear a lecture about nutrition. He apologizes. Perhaps he will be more gentle with the next woman with breast cancer whom he meets.

I welcome my anger at the lead-a-pure-life theorists. I consider it a step toward my healing. I try to be conscious of my diet and lifestyle, in order to give my body every advantage. Of course the mind and body are interrelated. We can regulate our lifestyles toward good health. Can we do so in a way to prevent breast cancer? No one knows. No one knows the cause of breast cancer. No one knows the cure.

Vegetarians and yoga teachers die of breast cancer, as do meat eaters and tap water drinkers. Breast cancer finds confident women as readily as it does those who are meek. Tumors come to both the sunny and the depressed.

Variation #3:
Cancer as Repressed Anger

I am having lunch in a San Francisco café with a therapist who leads a breast cancer support project. She uses movement to help women learn to feel comfortable in their bodies, which have been assaulted by cancer, surgery, and adjuvant treatments. I am interested in the connection between the arts and healing and find her work intriguing.

Then, she begins to talk about the personality types of women with breast cancer and of the repressed-anger-causes-breast-cancer theory. I cannot believe my ears. She really believes this stuff. An enlightened therapist? In California? Oh no, anything but this. I consider bopping her on the head with my salad fork. She must rush off. I am sorry we did not have more time together. I will make time in the future. Before she reinforces this idea in the women who are trying to heal.

❧

My diagnosis sent me rushing to my university's medical library. The dreaded graduate course in statistics proved invaluable. I know how to read quantitative research. I looked at study after study and found no causal link between breast cancer and diet. Or to weight. Or to wine. Or to personality type. Or emotions. Or to repressed anger.

What protected me from self-blame? After my diagnosis, I could not stand to read self-help books. But I began to read biology. I was swept up in the sheer miracle of the life and death cycles of organisms. Here, right inside my body, were these ancient forces, optimized to their environment over millions of years. More than any advice or medical prognosis, this realization comforted me. My body's cellular wisdom operates day and night, with or without my awareness. Knowledge of medicine or psychology or diet can prolong life, but this knowledge is minuscule compared to the miracle of life itself.

My second protection was my spiritual practice. I did not experience the calm and clarity that I had imagined in a crisis. I lived in a volcano of emotions. I often had no idea what to do. Yet in ways I had not imagined, I was prepared.

My meditation training comes from the tradition of the Sufis. One of the foundational practices, handed down from teacher to student for hundreds of years, is called "remembrance." This meditation is done with gentle motions, sound, and breath, which focus concentration and involve the body as well as the mind. Making a circle with my head, I sweep away my limited point of view, like a broom sweeping away cobwebs. This practice, which means "There is nothing except God," is repeated many times, much like the Jesus prayer of the early Christian monks. It begins with a word which means "No."

Thousands of times in my meditation, I practice saying "No." At the end of each repetition, the breath is held for a few moments in silent contemplation of the divine presence.

This practice is done on retreat, or during periods of daily meditation. It offers no promises of material benefits or guarantees of success. It is designed to allow a direct experience of the sacredness of this world, which is so easily overlooked or forgotten. That is why the practice is called *remembrance*. Life, whether in suffering or joy, becomes a most holy place.

Much like the psychological development of the child, saying "No" is an early lesson of spiritual development. It is the core of discernment in both action and thought, requiring intense examination of beliefs and motivations. "Going with the flow" is a mistaken image of meditation. Because it is often easier to say "Yes," the power of "No" takes patience and courage.

When meditation reaches the psyche, the practice begins to work in life. This gentle, persistent "No" questions assumptions about self-worth, perfection, failure, and the fine line between responsibility and what is beyond our control. As the "No" chips away old patterns, it opens space for fresh insights. It acts as a wedge against automatic thinking, against thoughts such as, "If I have breast cancer, it *must* be my fault." This is an assumption, a speculation. Why must it be my fault? Why aren't other explanations just as plausible? Why pick self-blame as the #1 option?

I discovered laughter as an antidote to my tendency toward guilt, a personal habit and heritage of my upbringing. My daughter and I collapsed in giggles because I felt guilty about not finishing a book about what is wrong with guilt. I found delight in accepting that I was not perfect.

I do not know how to eradicate cancer, but perhaps I can help eradicate the dark thoughts of guilt and blame for a disease with an unknown cause. I am working with my surgeon to write new orientation materials for the Breast Center where I was treated. He sees many patients who fear that they have created their cancer. In a letter, which could be addressed to any woman, this surgeon/researcher says, "If I must tell you that you have breast cancer, please remember that it is just one of those things that happens. Nobody wants you to have cancer."

Can we leave behind the thicket of the "if onlys"? Can we spare ourselves the torture of self-blame? Gather us up as exemplars: the meditator, the vegetarian, the assertive, and the physically fit. Yes, we have breast cancer. As do hundreds of thousands of women in all kinds of shapes and with all kinds of personal issues and habits. It is not our fault. Please wish us well. Did we create this? Are we to blame for our breast cancer? This question is an open invitation to spiritual practice. Anyone can do this meditation. It is the sacred practice of "No."

Karen

When I was first diagnosed, I spent a lot of time trying to figure out what I had done wrong that would give me cancer. There is absolutely no history of breast cancer in my family, so it *must* have been something I, personally did. But the scientific evidence would not give me the satisfaction of pinpointing a single cause. I had smoked for several years, but the link between smoking and breast cancer is tenuous at best. I carried around a few extra pounds but, according to the literature, that didn't really seem to make a huge difference. I was thirty-six and had never given birth—that raised my chances an infinitesimal amount. All that musing was finally put to rest when an oncology nurse said to me, "As far as the causes of cancer go, there is one apparent fact and a lot of guesses. Cigarette smoking appears to cause lung cancer. After that, the main cause of cancer is life."

So maybe it was environmental. I have never been a big one for washing my produce. As long as I could not see the dirt, it was clean enough for me. Who knew what level of carcinogenic pesticide I had built up inside my body? Or maybe it was the "mosquito trucks," puffing out huge clouds of what I later figured out was DDT, that used to come around the neighborhood where I lived in Florida as a child. Then again, I *did* take a tour of Three Mile Island once—post-disaster. Or I remembered that my father had given me one of his childhood souvenirs: a radioactive dime from some science museum. That thing was probably still in one of my memento boxes. But if one of these things was the cause, why have there not been epidemics of breast cancer in tropical areas, or in TMI tour groups?

Well, maybe it was not something I did *physically*. More and more evidence is pouring in suggesting that our psychological state has effects on our physical health. I went through a terrible depression when I got divorced. Maybe that was it. Or that heartbreaking relationship that ended in 1992. That would have been about two years before I was diagnosed, and they say the majority of people who are diagnosed with cancer have had a major stressor in their lives in the previous two years. But then I read something by author and breast cancer patient Jory

Graham: how good it would be if only we *had* created our cancers psychologically. Then an excellent psychiatrist could cure us.

Whatever the cause, I went through my lumpectomy and six weeks of radiation. I endured six rounds of the chemotherapy regimen CAF. Then I had a party to say good-bye to cancer, and was just about ready to go without my wig when I went for my first two-month checkup. The news was not good: the cancer had metastasized, and I had tumors in my lungs. By that point, I had read enough to know what this meant: I was Stage IV, and terminal. I wailed to my physician: "But I've done everything right! I've taken all my treatments, and I've kept a positive attitude, and... and...." She nodded. "Yes, you've been very compliant."

It was then I realized I had spent eight months searching for what I had done wrong because there was only one alternative: I had not caused this cancer. And if I had not caused it, then that meant I was not in control and *that* meant I could not cure myself. Suddenly I was abandoned to the chaos of the universe.

Of course, all the time I was asking these epidemiological questions, I was also having quite a conversation with God. "Why me?" I asked. What did *I* do to deserve this? I am not a saint, but I am a decent person. I felt like King Lear: I was more sinned against than sinning. Then one day the "Why me?" turned around and became, "Why *not* me?" Each year there are millions of children in this world who die before they reach their first birthdays. Millions of innocent Jews died during the Holocaust. Who was I to be exempt?

There was only one problem with these lines of thought, both the scientific and religious: taken together they laid my cancer at the feet of God. Some of my more conservative Christian friends urged me to consider what I was being punished for. Some of my New Age friends told me there was a spiritual reason behind my cancer, and my task was to find it.

I have never believed in a vindictive God. The New Testament story that disturbs me the most is when God strikes down Ananias and Sapphira because they have not been honest about their contributions to the church. I have occasionally questioned whether God loves me in particular, but that she loves every single human being I have never doubted. So I simply could not believe that God was either punishing me for something I had done or was using this terrible disease to teach me a lesson I should have caught in Sunday School.

Over the past four years there have been two passages of Scripture I have read hundreds of times. The first is the story of Job. He was a righteous man who suffered because of a little side bet God had going with Satan. His friends tried to convince him that he was suffering because of something he had done, but even Yahweh quashes that idea when he appears at the end of the book. The other Scripture that has grabbed on to me and not let go is the story of Jesus' passion. Another righteous man suffering innocently. And, after all, as the Gospel of Matthew says, the rain falls alike on the just and the unjust.

That is very helpful, because while I do not believe I "deserved" my cancer, I know I am not a righteous woman. My suffering can never be completely innocent, the way Jesus' or Job's was. But it is also true that there is no correlation between what I have suffered and the wrongs I have done. Today, I think there is a reason that I and others are so prone to blame the patient for the cancer. I have always been the responsible type, with a superego big enough to make any psychoanalyst salivate. I like to believe I am in charge of my life. I like to believe I get out of life what I put into it. If I eat well—say no more than twenty-five grams of fat a day—I assume I will stay well and will never have cancer. If I exercise right—say minimally twenty minutes three times a week—I assume I will not get sick, and certainly will never have cancer. But there is a flaw in that line of thought. What does it have to say about the twenty-four-year-old aerobics instructor in my support group who has breast cancer? How about my brother-in-law, the health nut? He has, since his youth, eaten only the best foods and exercised like a madman. And yet he was diagnosed with testicular cancer. He is well now, thank God, but he wears a T-shirt that says, "Eat right. Exercise. Die anyway."

Death is perhaps the ultimate evidence that I am not in control of my own life. Given reasonable mental and physical health and freedom from pain, I do not know anyone who would want to die. And yet it happens to each of us.

Christianity has always promoted the doctrine of *creation ex nihilo,* the idea that God made creation out of absolutely nothing. The vocabulary in the first chapter of Genesis, though, suggests that God made order out of chaos. The natural state of the universe, and our lives, is chaos. It is only through the action of God that there is any order at all. That includes creation, and it includes health. If it were not for God's action in our world, we would all have cancer.

Again, though, this leaves my cancer at the feet of God. I do not believe, as some of my friends do, that God *caused* my cancer. I do not believe that God works like the Gary Larsen "Far Side" cartoon that shows God punching the "Smite" key at a computer, while the monitor shows an unsuspecting man about to meet his death by a falling piano.

On the other hand, if I believe in a God who is all-good and all-powerful (and I do), I must also believe that if God did not *cause* my cancer, she certainly *permitted* it. This is where things get scary. I would rather blame myself for my cancer than face these questions about God. What kind of God allows women to get breast cancer? What kind of God creates human beings in such a way that to be a woman means estrogen can suddenly change from friend to enemy? What kind of God sends a male savior who cannot understand the first thing about having breast cancer? What kind of God creates a world in which every living thing eventually dies?

It is hard for me not to picture God as a huge, all-powerful Karen, stripped of sin and psychopathology. It is tempting for me to say, "If *I* were God, I would *never* let women get breast cancer. I would *never* let anyone die." I cannot imagine how it can be that I am more compassionate than God.

And here I draw close to the reason I would rather blame myself than God for my cancer. If God is good and yet allows cancer and death, then it must be that God is "good" in a way I cannot even begin to understand. God is not just a big, powerful Karen. God is apparently not like the pictures drawn by any of the contemporary theologians I have ever read. In looking through the lens of eternity, that unfamiliar God may see that my cancer is, indeed, "good." Perhaps that strange God allowed my cancer to develop for a particular reason. I cannot understand it at all. I do believe that one day, on the other side of death, I will understand.

This God I have discovered is not very likeable. She is much wilder than the God I always met in Sunday School and church, tied up in a neat little package labeled "God is love." Love, all right. But can it be loving to allow me, her daughter, to have breast cancer? Along with that question, though, I have to ask myself if it can be loving to allow Jesus, her son, to die on the cross.

Living with breast cancer has torn me away from the God I used to know and initiated me into the priesthood of a very different God. This God is bigger, less understandable, less like me, more concerned with my eternal life as a whole than my misery of the moment. This is a God of mystery. As I said, I do not know that I *like* her very much. But I passionately love her.

Many of my friends are horrified by the God I have come to know. But I love her, first and foremost, because she takes the job of being God away from me. She is so different from me that I know I cannot control the world, my life. She is so involved in my day-to-day life and yet so grounded in eternity that she knows with absolute certainty what is good for me in my life as a whole. I love this God, too, because she is compassionate. I know she loathes my suffering. I know because she became a human being and experienced what it is like to suffer. I know she has given me tremendous gifts in the midst of my cancer, and I know that she has given me this odd, long "normal" time between a terminal diagnosis and death.

Since my original diagnosis, I have always had plenty of people willing to help me figure out whether I caused my cancer. When I meet and get to know someone new, it almost always comes up. I finally came to understand why this happens. If my new friend can pinpoint the cause of my cancer, then that means she can avoid that cause and keep herself safe. To believe that, even unconsciously, is easier than recognizing the essential chaos in our world and our own vulnerability.

The creation of my cancer is not my major concern these days. Perhaps that is because I am four years out from my diagnosis. Maybe it is because I face death every day, and my thoughts automatically move to larger questions and longer spans of time. So the short answer to the direct question of whether I created my cancer is this: "I don't know. Probably." But the considered answer, the one I have given here, has to be, "No. I am not God."

Linda

Who knows when cancer begins, and why; our knowledge often comes long after cancer has invaded our bodies.

For me, the first hint came in the summer of 1992. I was painting my living room, and I pushed up my T-shirt to wipe the sweat that was reminding me it was August in the South, where, as usual, it wasn't the heat, it was the humidity. The edge of my hand slid across my chest, and I felt a hard lump where the curve of my left breast smoothed out toward my breastbone.

It's only in the movies that at such a moment the response is dramatic and philosophical. Vivien Leigh would have swooned gracefully, Bette Davis would have stormed out of the room, a ribbon of cigarette smoke trailing behind her. But me? I sat down hard on the couch and said, "Oh, shit."

Quickly, though, I remembered: "I had a mammogram in June, two months ago. So it must be nothing, right?"

Wrong.

It was not "nothing," although it took a few months to discover that.

In a couple of weeks I saw an internist and she recommended I see a surgeon. In a couple more weeks I met with a surgeon and we talked about possibilities. Yes, it could be a tumor, but it was more likely just normal changes in breast tissue. I was, after all, peri-menopausal and several years earlier had had benign cysts removed from both breasts.

And the mammogram—the screening that may save millions of lives by early detection—showed nothing abnormal.

So I went home and "watched" the lump, a phrase that hardly describes what I actually did. Every day I touched it, I moved my fingertips over it without any pain or real sensation. It was small and hard, almost like some bizarre bone spur that would not have been out of the ordinary on my middle-aged knees, but instead appeared on my chest.

Six months passed. In February, just after my forty-fourth birthday and just before a scheduled follow-up with the surgeon, when I wasn't even "watching" it—I was taking a shower—I felt something very different. It was bigger. Maybe harder. Yes, definitely harder.

My reaction, still undramatic, was ungrammatical but accurate: "This ain't right."

Two days later, the surgeon examined the lump that had changed so quickly. She agreed with my assessment, although she was more professional and articulate.

There were phone calls to day surgery and pathology, appointments for pre-op X rays and blood tests, and an hour later I left the doctor's office. The calendar I clutched in my hand showed a week that already included three interviews for newspaper stories for my job as a feature writer, lunch with my boss, and a birthday party.

Now there was an addition for 9 A.M. Friday, March 5, 1993: "Saint Thomas/biopsy."

It was to be an excisional biopsy—the surgeon would remove all of the mass if possible, not just a sample.

I kept that appointment, and three hours later, in the recovery room, the surgeon leaned over the rail of my bed.

"This is a cancer," she said. "I'm sorry."

It was a moment before I realized she was speaking again. "Mastectomy ... chemotherapy ... radiation."

"What day is it?" I asked her.

"March 5th."

"I guess I won't be going to Spain on the 28th."

Instead my journey would be to a place in my heart where I had not gone before, might never have gone if cancer had not taken me there.

It is a journey that each of us makes in her own way. For me, it was important to travel light.

How do you do that when the burden is one that society has long deemed heavy? Only a few years ago, the word *cancer* was not even spoken by those who were living—and dying—with it. There was for many a blanket of shame, a shadow of guilt, or a weight of responsibility.

I was spared that because the foundation of my spirituality, anchored in a recovery program that millions know as "The Twelve Steps," is one of acceptance. It is an assurance that there are no mistakes in God's world, that everything is as it should be right now.

Before you think, "What a Pollyanna!" let me say that when things are moving along according to God's plan for my life, I don't necessarily like it. "Everything is as it should be" is by no means the same thing as "Everything is coming up roses." When breast cancer arrived, I did not welcome it, but I did accept it.

And, yes, I wondered what it was doing there. A newspaper reporter for more than twenty-five years, I was in an environment where I was exposed to reports of risk factors and research efforts and medical advances in many areas, breast cancer among them.

If I'd wanted to—if I wanted to today—I could provide a fact sheet of my life that would include many things that might have contributed to my cancer. I had no full-term pregnancies. I abused alcohol and other drugs for many years. Extra pounds slowly added to my frame until, when I was forty years old, I was also forty pounds overweight. I grew up in the Deep South, and annually ate nearly my weight in red meat. I exercised sporadically. I worked very hard in a high-stress profession. Depression had stalked me since childhood.

But did I cause my cancer? I don't think so. Did the pollutants in the air and water of the highly industrialized Tennessee River town where I spent half my life cause it? No. Did my genetic heritage—three maternal aunts with breast cancer and my mother's lymphoma—cause it? No.

All of those factors, of course, may have played a part for me, as they may have for thousands of other women who face breast cancer and other illnesses. Still, blaming heredity or environment or one's personal choices, however poor they might be, neither advances the spiritual journey nor promotes healing in body or soul.

I can only say to others, as I have to myself, that I believe we arrive in this life as spiritual beings, and one of our tasks here is to learn to be human. For me, cancer has been my greatest teacher and my greatest gift. In four difficult years following the diagnosis, my heart embraced a life lesson that Adrienne Rich shared in her poetry: "I came to see the damage that was done and the treasures that prevail."

Dignity, of course, is not one of those treasures. You move through all the pre-op tests, and you imagine that you'll create a sacred space to move into for the next phase of the journey, the one where you will, perhaps, give up a breast (or a piece of one, or both of them). Instead you find yourself filling your altar with Fleet enemas to use according to your pre-op instructions and accordion folders to keep up with your insurance claims.

Yes, at those times it's hard to remember that cancer is not a punishment for one's failures or excesses. But a lesson in humility? Yes, and that's one of the treasures that prevails.

En route to the hospital for the next step, a mastectomy, I turned to the friend who was driving and said, "This is really not what I want to do today." I would say the same thing two months later as we waited to begin my first chemotherapy treatment.

But, each time, the resistance was momentary. I had surrendered my illusion of control, tossed it over into the heap reserved for guilt and shame and fear.

With a rough map of a route that was remote from anything I had ever known, I began the journey. For about an hour, I was in a hospital room with my friend and my therapist, the two women I'd asked to be there. I needed them to save my life, for that day and days and months to come; they did, with so much love and acceptance that even now when I think of it the tears come in a hot flood. I asked a hundred questions:

"Did you get a room at the lodge for my parents?"

"Are you sure someone is taking care of my cat?"

"Am I going to get through this?"

The answers were always "Yes," but when I was taken away from that room, wheeled down endless corridors, and prepared for surgery, getting through it seemed remote. I wanted to cry, but I feared that if I started I might never stop.

In the operating room there were so many people, and they were all very busy. I lay on my back, drowsy, but cold and frightened and alone, even though I was the center of attention. The lights were so bright.

Go to sleep, go to sleep. And when you wake up your life will be changed forever. You may lose your breast, then your hair, and your dignity from time to time, but you can fill in the gaps from a deep well of courage and strength. That is not necessarily a bad deal.

Chaos

THE SHOCK OF DIAGNOSIS STARTS A PROCESS of disintegration. Will God help or am I on my own? Does death mean I lose? Does God get to vote? Whom should I tell? This is the stage of facing our own death. It is also a test of our relationship with a power greater than ourselves. What can be done to support a woman in this stage? Resist the urge to say, "Everything will be all right." It may not be. Although cancer is not synonymous with death, people do die from this disease. Facing death is a life wish, not a death wish.

> *If a man wishes to be sure of the road he treads on,*
> *he must close his eyes and walk in the dark.*
> —SAINT JOHN OF THE CROSS

The prevalent terminology that speaks of breast cancer survivors as "winners" reveals a darker flip side: Those who are more immediately facing death are often viewed as "losers." But can we go beyond that either/or thinking, can we see death not as "losing"?

Many of us who get breast cancer are faced with terrifying decisions about treatment: Do I have the right doctor? Should I go to another city for a second opinion? Should I just have a lumpectomy? Should I have mastectomies on both my breasts? We soon discover that the medical establishment is of some help, but often turns important questions back to us to answer. How do we make the best decisions for ourselves?

To face cancer or other life-threatening illnesses, we need a new spiritual response to choices and decision making as well as to death and dying. We want to live deeper, richer lives, not despite the fact that we all someday will die, but because of the preciousness such awareness brings.

Does Death Mean I Lose?

Carol

After your illness becomes publicly known, this funny thing happens to the greetings of many acquaintances: Their eyes fix deeply into yours, their hands grasp yours tightly, and they say, "How are you?"—the *are* stretching two full beats. The thing is, even though I appreciated their genuine concern for me, I often felt a peculiar discomfort from the ritual exchange. Gradually I began to understand that because of my brush with mortality, I had crossed an unspoken threshold. From an outsider's perspective, I had fallen into the enemy's hands. Mixed with the compassion of their ritual words and gestures were unexpressed feelings of helplessness and terror in the face of death, the enemy.

On my side of the line, however, I was coming to terms with death not as an enemy, but as a natural part of life's rhythm. I could feel it in my gut for the first time that life really does come in limited quantities for every one of us. To whatever degree I had previously taken life for granted, I was now treasuring the gift of time for however long I had left. There is great irony in this. On the other side of the threshold, many of my greeters viewed death as the destroyer of meaning. But on my side of the line, I began to see it as exactly the opposite. Death is, in truth, not the destroyer but rather the creator of meaning.

For instance, between my first and second rounds of chemotherapy, it suddenly became very important to me to get Dan and the kids to help me paint the kitchen. With my hair having just fallen out, I think they would have done anything for me. But what I wanted was a painted kitchen. Tan. So there we were, the four of us wearing old baseball caps, splattered with paint, working to the beat of the Beatles blasting from the boom box. Toward the end of the weekend, we were standing back admiring our work when I inexplicably burst into tears. Not knowing what was wrong, my family huddled around me until I could finally choke out what was going on. You see, I had been overwhelmed by my love for them—and the love had come bundled with incredible sadness over how much I would miss being with them if I died. In truth, my love was so strong, I felt like I was burning up inside. I was like the Seraphim in the Jewish tradition, angels in attendance to God whose only job is to recite "Holy, Holy, Holy" three times. The thing is, the passion of their emotion is so great, they can only get partway through the first holy before burning up with love.

Long before I could put words to what I was experiencing, I was having spontaneous combustions of this nature on a fairly regular basis. This is not to say, however, that I never fell prey to major bouts of self-pity, sure that I was some kind of big-time loser singled out by God for special punishment. How could I not? After all, we live in a society of people who are fascinated by death—as long as it is on the TV news or in the movie theaters—but who are terrified of their own mortality. We purchase expensive cosmetics and undergo surgery to stave off signs of aging, a reminder of our final destination. In our real lives, we want people's deaths to be antiseptic and out of sight, handled somewhere off-stage by designated institutions and professionals.

I knew from my spiritual studies that other cultures handle death better than we do in the West. Many societies deeply value their old people, honoring their wisdom and accepting their deaths as the culmination rather than the destruction of their long, rich lives. Eastern mystics meditate in graveyards in order to stay conscious of the transitory nature of existence. And even now in the West there are signs of a grassroots recovery from the age of rationality, with an increasing number of people in both mainstream religion and the New Age who take comfort and meaning from spiritual beliefs about reincarnation and the afterlife.

Thankfully, when I felt singled out in my misfortune, I did not suffer silently. From the beginning, I was in active conversation with God about my illness. On second thought, conversation is, perhaps, too polite a word. I yelled at God. I cried. I negotiated. I begged. I wheedled and prayed. Happily, in the Jewish tradition, the Scriptures are filled with role models who held nothing back from their relationships with God: Moses begging God to pick somebody else to be God's voice on earth; Abraham heatedly negotiating with God to save Sodom for the few righteous people; Jacob wrestling with God's agent at the banks of the Jabbok River, demanding that God give him a blessing.

Often my dialogue with God was only in my mind, expressed in wordless yearning colored by shades of despair. But sometimes, I sat down to work through my feelings in my daily journal. One day, when I was at my lowest, I asked God point blank how scaring me so badly could possibly be part of a divine plan for me. Hadn't I done my part to be a good enough person? I began to write my questions down for God. Amazed, I watched as God used my pen to reply.

> G (GOD): You know, Carol, you are so narrowly focused on the issue of whether you are going to live or die. You are missing the point. You must understand, there are worse things than dying.
>
> C (CAROL): Like what?
>
> G: Like letting the forces of darkness dim your light.
>
> C: How do they do that?
>
> G: By having you doubt yourself and lose faith in me, believing that the darkness is right about you.
>
> C: It's not?

G: What is happening to you has nothing to do with who you are and how I feel about you. Think about it for a minute: If dying means you lose, then everybody's a loser.

C: It's possible to die and not be a loser?

G: How could you ask such a question? You know the story of Rabbi Akiba. Rather than recant his belief in me, he was tortured to death. Even as the pain consumed his body, he died with the Sh'ma on his lips. He didn't die a loser—he died a free man. When a person steps forward in the power of their light, they don't just do it for themselves, but for all humanity.

C: You want me to be a martyr?

G: You do not want to be a martyr, and neither did he. What you do want is to stand firm in my light no matter what. You do not focus on the results. Rather, you focus on your sacred task: living fully in the holy present, regardless of the circumstances you face.

C: But why does it have to be so painful? If you sent me breast cancer as some kind of lesson or test, you must know it could kill me!

G: Freedom is my greatest gift, but you pay the price of having to wrestle with your fear. Remember, when you stand up to the darkness, you do it for all humanity.

C: And if I die first?

G: You die free.

C: But God, I don't want to die. I love my life.

G: That is the ultimate paradox. Unless you truly understand the preciousness of life, you can't be truly free.

C: But the fear spoils it. Fear of loss, of pain.

G: Then give up the fear.

C: How do I give up the fear?

G: By having faith.

C: Simple for you to say. Harder to do. But maybe I could take some comfort in believing that you have some greater purpose in mind for me, regardless of what happens to me.

G: No, not regardless... *because* of whatever happens. I am asking you to face your fate courageously, with trust and faith and no regret, no matter what the outcome may be. Be willing to do that, and you will have done all that I've asked of you. You will have made a difference.

For many years, when I thought of fulfilling my human potential, I thought only of attaining more control over my life—of peace and happiness for myself. After this dialogue with God, I realized how narrow was the band of life's experiences I had set out to achieve. Now I understand that to be truly alive is to expand and embrace the broader range of human experience: bittersweet sadness, righteous anger, even deep and honest despair. I surrender the illusion that this is my show. I allow my heart to break open. It is through the cracks that God enters and stirs my heart and soul to their fullest expression. This is the true fulfillment of one's human potential, and it comes only when you are willing to let your own self-reliant spirit be broken.

Susan

I thought I was ready for death. After all, the thought of death is part of my daily spiritual practice. The mystical imagery of my Sufi tradition is filled with quotes from dervishes who say, "Die before death and live forever!" Or the words of poets like Rumi who say, "Now you must be annihilated in love." This is the good kind of death, the death of what the mystics call the false self. The old self is supposed to shatter like an eggshell, making room for a new self, one that is made in the image of God. This transformation is the essence of the spiritual path.

Then I heard the words: *You have cancer.* The translation in my mind and body was immediate and visceral. "I am going to die." There was nothing the least bit spiritual about this experience. Oh, no, not *this* kind of death. This death of the body, good-bye, never enjoy the air or a kiss, an endless nothing kind of death. I was not centered or mystical. I was in shock.

One out of three people gets cancer. My brother-in-law was diagnosed with brain cancer six months before I learned I had breast cancer. He lived less than two years past that day, and his determination to live never waned. We talked often during this time. Although his diagnosis was much more grave than mine, our first reactions were surprisingly similar. The initial shock of a life-threatening disease is intense. The mind leaps to the next question: "How long do I have to live?"

No one knows. Statistics predict the chances of getting and surviving a given disease. I once heard a description of these statistics, that they are stories without tears. The statistics were my reality. I never felt like a victim. Even with my family history, it seemed like a random throw of the dice. I had drawn the short straw.

I never felt as if I were in battle with my disease. My struggle was for understanding. My deepest feeling throughout my illness was a sense of loss, but not the "I lose" of a fight. Mine was the loss associated with grief, and the loss of a sense of well-being that I took for granted. I felt that my body had betrayed me. My only other major illness was much different than my cancer diagnosis. I had almost died when our son was born. Yet I was not then plunged into the dark fear of death evoked by cancer.

I had toxemia in my first pregnancy. For some reason, the baby poisons the mother's body, and in response, her blood pressure rises to alarming levels, which can cause a stroke. The doctors told me I had one of the most severe cases they had ever seen. They taped a tongue depressor on the wall by my hospital bed so someone could clear my airway when I had the expected seizure.

This disease was perhaps more life-threatening than my cancer. But in this crisis, I did not believe I was going to die. Three factors kept this thought away. One was my conclusion that the doctors were idiots. Their frenetic pace and misreading of clinical tests sharply contrasted my blissful state of pregnancy.

Second, I was graced during this period with an extraordinary intuitive clarity. I knew when to consent to procedures and when to protest. My decisions turned out to be correct. My body was at death's door, but not my mind. I left the hospital against doctor's orders. Back in my own surroundings, my blood pressure returned to normal. I had my second baby at home. That was my last encounter with the serious side of medicine until I found myself in the surgeon's examining room, about to learn that I had cancer.

The third reason that I did not equate my toxemia with death was that I had never heard of anyone dying of it. Because of prenatal care, it is no longer a major cause of death for women in childbirth. This is not the same for cancer. Cancer is our modern-day version of the plague. The word itself evokes fear. This fear is heightened by constant news from the front about medical research, the "war on cancer." There is much progress, but the death rate, especially for advanced metastatic disease, stays about the same.

Illness has very different effects on the body, the mind, and the spirit. These effects may be related, or independent of one another. My toxemia was life-threatening, but I had little fear; my prognosis from cancer was excellent, yet I was convinced I was about to die. My emotions were a tangle. The intuition that I was given during my first illness was gone.

The thought of death continues to be part of my meditation practice, but I am much more humble in claiming that I understand. I am so glad to be alive that having a false ego is not high on my list of worries. Cancer turned out to be a spiritual catalyst. Something I had been sensing for years became concrete. It is hard to put into words. Maybe it is the experience of the spirit made into flesh. Life is borrowed and exquisitely precious.

I don't know if I will ever say that I have come to terms with cancer. I view it as a chronic disease, something that may recur, or may be present though undetected. I do not think about it every day. It is fading into the background, becoming something else that can happen to me.

I hold in my heart all those with great spirit and determination, people like my brother-in-law, who die of cancer. Or people like Carol's friend who died of lung cancer, an effervescent woman who worried that her fighting efforts were not good enough.

Some research studies suggest that a "fighting spirit" may prolong life. Whether or not this is true, it does not guarantee a cure. The concept of "fighting spirit" has a dark side, especially when we say some-one "lost her battle." It leaves open that terrible door to believing that if she had fought harder, she would still be alive.

There are other, more positive, metaphors for disease. The poet Rumi writes that being a person is like being a guesthouse. Joy, depres-sion, illness, and fear come as unexpected visitors. Our job is to welcome every guest, even if they are a crowd of sorrows. Each may be a guide to some further understanding.

If I die of cancer, I do not want my obituary to say, "She lost her battle with cancer." Instead, please write, "She welcomed every guest." And that she lived—and died—in the best way she knew how.

Karen

There was a time when my oncologist suggested I might have only six months to live. Luckily, he found a treatment that has put me into an odd sort of "remission" that has continued for two and a half years, as I am writing this. Neither he nor I has any idea how long this will last. And despite my apparent health today, the fact still remains: I am ter-minally ill.

I was on a panel at a local hospital's conference when one of the speakers tried to console me: "After all, I could get hit by a truck this afternoon," she said. My response was, "I'll trade ya." What people do not seem to realize is that I have *already* been hit by a truck, a truck called "cancer," and my life is at stake.

I seem to get two reactions to my terminal prognosis. One is the people who, like the woman at the conference, try to tell me my cancer is really no big deal. There are so many people who have it worse than me, they tell me. This is true, but knowing that fact does not at all lighten my burden. In fact, just the opposite.

"Cheer up," they say, and "You're going to be just fine, I know it." I cannot cheer up because I am not in a cheery situation. I know in my heart that people say these sorts of things because they are concerned for me. They do not like to think of the bad possibilities any more than I do. They are reassuring themselves as much as me that I am going to be all right. The problem is that all the reassurance in the world does not change reality. They can make my cancer a tiny little thing in their minds, but I still have to live with it in its full strength, and part of that reality is death.

The other reaction, the one I encounter more often, is utter, unconscious horror. I will never forget running into a professor not long after my surgery. He asked how I was doing, and as I was telling him, I noticed he moved away from me. I was not hearing a word he was saying; all I could do was listen to his body language. I decided to test him. I took a step toward him, and he moved two steps back. I waited a few minutes and did it again. Every time, the same thing happened. He simply could not stand to be near me. It is as if I have the words *You are going to die* tattooed on my forehead, and people do not like looking at me because I remind them of their mortality.

One of my darkest times was when I was given that six-month estimate. I had been diagnosed in April 1994; in December of that year, my cancer metastasized. I was enrolled in a clinical trial and a few months later, I had new tumors. At that point, all of medical science had not found anything that would touch my cancer, and so I heard "Six months." That very same day, my fiancé left me. He said as he went, "You're probably going to die soon, and I have to get away so it doesn't hurt so much."

He was not the first person in my life to leave because of the cancer. My closest woman friend, a Lutheran minister, was attentive at first but became more and more remote. We were used to talking on the phone a couple of times a day, and going to dinner once a week or so. Her calls stopped, as did our time together. I confronted her—twice. Both times she wept and threw up her hands. I saw her recently at a mutual acquaintance's retirement dinner, and after we spoke I realized it was the first time in over two years.

I was complaining to my minister about all of this once, and he asked me if I were not just catastrophizing. So I sat and wrote down the names of all the friends who had disappeared from my life since my diagnosis. There were twenty-six names on that list. Some were closer than others, both geographically and emotionally, and some hung in there longer than others. But they all disappeared sooner or later. Twenty-six.

The reason, of course, is that I remind people they are going to die. This is not a popular sentiment in American culture. People really seem to believe that if they eat enough broccoli and exercise enough, they will live forever. And I was only thirty-six when I was diagnosed; most people that age do not think of death very often.

I found myself aggravated and then angry as I read more and more of the popular cancer literature. Magazines seemed to profile only women who had recovered from Stage I or Stage II breast cancer. I do not want to minimize the horror of even the earliest diagnosis—cancer is awful whenever it happens. But the fact was that no one, not even the "cancer people," wanted to look at the women who were going to die— and that meant me.

I even felt some shame about it. So often, people talked about their lives years in the future, and I sat there, almost embarrassed, as I realized I would not be around when these things happened. I am not, and can never be, one of the breast cancer "winners." I am Stage IV, I am terminal, I am a loser. Or so the language of our culture says, even the subculture of breast cancer.

I have a friend who is HIV-positive. He was lucky to be in the early clinical trials for protease inhibitors, and one day I asked him how he was doing. He told me his virus load was undetectable, and now, instead of figuring out how to die gracefully, he was having to think once again of how to live. And he said it even made him a little angry.

I understand what my friend means. The fact is that we all die. In American culture, when we think of death at all, we hope it will happen when we are ninety-three years old, while we sleep, the night before we are supposed to go to the nursing home. There is a cycle of life and aging that gives us time to get used to the idea of dying—children grow up, leave home, and have their own kids. Retirement comes along. Spouses and friends die. But to be called upon to make peace with death at age thirty-six is unusual.

I was in uncharted territory, really. I have learned many skills in my life before, but learning how to die was a difficult one. What I discovered was that the closer I came to accepting death, the more I loved life.

We take so much for granted, we middle-class Americans. When we push the fact of death to the back of our psyches, we deprive ourselves of a very important realization: Life is so very precious, precisely because we will all die. I found a rubber stamp of a dancing skeleton and used it on my letters until my friends begged me to stop. But that skeleton illustrates a magnificent truth. The more we allow ourselves to live with our deaths, the more vibrantly we live while alive.

When I was dying, I had some of the happiest days of my life. I was not in pain and while the chemotherapy was no fun, I did have good days. One of my biggest pleasures was taking a shower after each of my ninety-six-hour Taxol infusions. During those five days I had "spit baths," as my mother called them, and the first shower after I got my chemo unhooked was a sensuous, exhilarating experience. The feeling of having water run all over my body, from the top of my head to my feet, was like an epiphany.

Very often, I would be at dinner or some social event with friends, and I would zone out. They teased me about this, but what was going on was that I had pulled away from the immediacy of what was happening around me to realize how special it all was, how good it felt to laugh so hard my stomach hurt, how wonderful to have friends sharing the details of their lives.

One of the blessings of cancer is that it gave me fresh eyes for the beauty of the world. Healthy people walked right by a dogwood tree in full bloom while I stood entranced for a full five minutes, caught up in that impossible lace that decorated branches seemingly dead just a few weeks ago. People gave me strange looks as I stood at a tree and felt the soft pods like pussy willows that were growing there. Even in the middle of the city in the rain I found incredible beauty; I looked out the window of my urban apartment and saw a plain black wrought-iron stair railing, glistening with the rays of the streetlight caught in the rain that covered it.

A professor once discovered me sitting on a bench on campus with my eyes closed. "What are you doing?" he said, and I told him I was just feeling the wind in my hair. He sped off to his next appointment, certain, I have no doubt, that my remaining sanity had finally left me. But I did not have hair for a year and a half, so at that moment, I felt joy. I loved, and still love, the way it feels when I have been on a long, hard walk and my scalp sweats; then the wind comes along and cools the moisture there and my head tingles all over. I exult in a windy day, when my hair goes all different directions; it feels like Mother Nature is gently tugging at my roots. Sometimes I grab a lock of hair and pull, *hard:* See, it didn't some out! Or to have someone brush my hair . . . well, some ecstasies are too profound to speak about.

There was a time when I was very sick and I could not do much more than sit up in bed and stare out my window, and the world was reduced to what I could see between the buildings that framed mine. But it turned out there was action enough for several days. Robins built a nest in the tree outside my window and noisily chased off the witless mourning doves who blundered anywhere nearby. People parked their cars on the side street and walked to the restaurant down the road arm in arm: neat young men with precision haircuts and shirts ironed so expertly they had to have come from the cleaners; young women with a studied casual style, the sweater thrown over their shoulders just so, the ankle socks slouching to just the right degree. They held their heads high and sneered at the dumpy old woman who walked her three-legged dog, but they were so transparent to me I could see the fragility of their self-assurance. It was as if they came to stand underneath my window and tell me about how badly they wanted to impress the person they were with. I wanted to pat their hands, to comfort them, to tell them to enjoy this uncertainty before they become middle-aged like me.

So there were many gifts in dying and, like my friend who is HIV-positive, I struggled for a while with anger when it appeared I was going to live a while more. It is not at all that I did not or do not want to live. It is just that being in the process of dying gave me eyes to see so much that I missed before, and since I have returned to the land of the living, I have started missing those things again. "Good health" has become routine, and so I rush past spring like everyone else. Well, not like everyone else—never again. But not as I did when I was dying.

My experience does give me some peace when I contemplate the end that will come someday. I hope it is not pain-filled, and I hope it does not last too long, because I do not want to be a burden on anyone. But I look forward to having that sharpened eyesight again, to having the veil of trivia lifted so I can see and feel all the things that are important.

In the cancer world, I am a failure when I die. But I am most fundamentally a Christian woman, and so death—whatever its cause—is ultimately a cause for rejoicing and for feelings of victory. I imagine to myself that in heaven I will have that sharpened eyesight all the time. Given what awaits me in the process of dying and what will come afterward, how in the world can I say that death means I lose?

Linda

When I was growing up in the '60s, there was a song by Bob Dylan, "Paths of Victory," that found a place in my psyche and has remained.

It says that the rough road is hard to travel, but it becomes clearer as the journey goes on. And it does. That song has meant different things at different points in my life. It was a promise that assured me that the agony of adolescence was not permanent. It was an anthem that acknowledged the social ills of its time would, somehow, someday, give way to peace and love. And, finally, in my forties, it was a reminder that only by living one day at a time would I slow the pace enough truly to experience joy, to take it in delicious gulps as if it were the air that sustains life.

It is, of course, for without joy, life becomes mechanical and the prospect of our inevitable death fearful.

When facing a life-threatening illness, it is important to remember that it is death that you cannot control—and it is life that you can experience to the fullest. Sometimes it's a difficult message to hold on to, since society and technology often seem to be on the other side, demanding that you use every possible measure to stay alive at all costs, despite the fact that the costs—emotional, financial, and spiritual—can be very high.

In *The Arrogance of Humanism,* David Ehrenfeld suggests that our civilization has come to equate the value of life with "the mere avoidance of death." That is, he said, not only an empty goal but an impossible one. It also hampers the joy, even the thrills, we can find in living, even as life moves us toward death.

The thrills, particularly in the midst of painful illness and sometimes even more painful treatment, may not be of the roller-coaster variety. But a rocking chair by a window, with the sun warming your face, can provide moments of joy, time for contemplation, and total immersion in the life-force.

In my own experience during treatment for breast cancer, I remember a time after a particularly difficult round of chemotherapy when I became aware that I was looking at death from a different angle.

The fatigue, nausea, mouth sores, and bottoming-out blood counts were taking their toll. Lying in bed, I realized that I was becoming aware of my body in all of what I thought to be its weakness—I had an image of the life-force slowly flowing from my body.

"This must be what it feels like to die," I thought.

But in that thought I felt not loss, but reassurance. My spirit was stronger than my body. All I had to do was to trust, to stay in touch, to go with the flow—another dictum from the '60s that I have used both unwisely and well at various times. And so it was that I received another of the lessons that cancer offered—I released my future to the future. For me, I kept today. On my best days, I still do.

I believe that it is my task to be as conscious as possible, to recognize that while cancer is a part of my life, it is also a part of my death, for life and death cannot be separated. Throughout the span of our lives, there are comings and goings, some lengthy and spectacular, others brief and quiet.

With the diagnosis of a life-threatening illness, with the knowledge that one in four of us who have breast cancer will die from the disease, I had already taken a long look through that door. I cannot tell you that I was ready to walk through it that day, or in the days that immediately followed. The bounty that has come with time, however, has given me a different perspective.

While diagnosis and treatment did not lead to my literal death, they put an end to the life I was living, and I will always be grateful for that. Honest. With the mastectomy that stripped away not only my breast but also the top layer of my pectoral muscle, which had been grasped by tiny fingers of cancer, I was wounded and vulnerable.

Emotionally, I repeated the process, tearing away the shell that had protected me from painful feelings and putting me, raw and open, into the chaos that was my life. I had gone into surgery on a gurney and returned through the birth canal. Obviously, I was not going to die; I had yet to be born.

So, with scars crisscrossing my chest and running hip to hip, I began a journey toward the somewhat uncharted landscape of my emotions. What I found there was more understanding than I had anticipated, and I expect that you will, too.

I tried to be kind to myself, no chiding for having failed to go to the well sooner and plumb its depths. We do what we have to do, when we can. A life-threatening illness just nudges us—or kicks us in the butt if we don't get out of the way in time.

I began the process of sorting out what was already dead in my life and what was alive but in serious need of nurturing. Shortly after I began chemotherapy, I went on a weekend retreat with a therapy group that I had been part of for two years. In two days of intensive and gut-wrenching work, we took our old lives apart and spread the pieces out. We assessed, discarded, retrieved, and rearranged the fragments, large and small, of who we had been and who we had become.

In the same fashion, cancer repeated that process for me, posing the questions that I had, until then, failed to formulate or to answer. The answers then revealed that while I was not afraid to die, I was not prepared to die. I am not a practicing Christian, and my concerns were not that I had not taken steps toward ensuring my place in the next life, but that I was falling way short of what I could experience in this one. So, it was not death that would deal me a loss, but life—and only because I wasn't proactive.

I stopped worrying about whether I would, like my great-grandmother, live to be ninety-seven. I considered that I needed to live fully at forty-four, forty-five, forty-six ... today. I learned to embrace life and to enjoy it, to cherish it, but not to cling to it.

Life is not something that we can possess; it is only something that we can experience, sometimes luxuriate in, and, yes, even agonize about. Each phase is part of the cycle. And then comes death; the wheel keeps turning.

In *The Cancer Journals,* the late feminist poet Audre Lorde speaks for many: "What is there possibly left for us to be afraid of, after we have dealt face to face with death and not embraced it? Once I accept the existence of dying, as a life process, who can ever have power over me again?"

THREE

Does God Get to Vote?

Carol

Before I was diagnosed with cancer, I thought of myself as the kind of woman who could be counted on to rise to any occasion. But suddenly, seated on a cold metal table wrapped in a flimsy hospital gown, I found myself in critical conversations having to do with my life and death in which I was easily the least educated person on the subject in the room. Physicians who had decades of training, who read hundreds of journals, who participated in cutting-edge research, who flew around the world to exchange the latest findings with their peers, talked to me about types, stages, choices, risks, and controversies in medical language I had never before heard. I really tried to listen when the doctors laid out my various treatment options, but I simply could not give it my best attention. For all the while my brain was screaming, "You're going to die,

You're going to die!" (Thankfully, a friend advised me to audiotape key sessions with my physicians so that I could listen to what was really said later.)

I had to make decisions and I had to make them fast. There were two obvious ways to go. I could try to climb back on top by hitting the medical library and the Internet, playing catch-up with the professionals. However, I trusted that my physicians were not only among the finest in their fields of expertise, but also that they truly had my best welfare at heart. Second-guessing them, particularly since I had not cracked open a science book since my early college days, seemed to be not the wisest use of my time. On the other hand, I could go limp and let the doctors tell me what I should do. That would have been a legitimate option if the choices I faced were clear-cut and not as personal as so many turned out to be.

One of the first things the cancer patient discovers is that very few of the choices that are presented come in black and white. There are competing theories, studies, and procedures. How much to cut away? How aggressive to be? Which course of treatment to undergo? Could a doctor decide for me whether I should take the risk of getting involved with a clinical trial of a new, unproved drug? Can a doctor decide whether I would be happier in the long run with or without reconstructive surgery? Can a doctor tell me whether to supplement or replace traditional treatment with an alternative?

Cancer has this funny way of cutting through all the superficial stuff that fills most of our days to get down to the rock-bottom issues—and fast. We think we are being asked to make scientific decisions about medical procedures. But the truth is, the questions that we are really being asked to answer are things like: How badly do I want to live? How important is physical beauty to me? How strong is my faith? My willingness to endure pain? What's my life about?

You can talk to the top experts in the field, make monumental lists of benefits versus risks, wring your brain dry trying to force out a rational solution, and be not one inch closer to knowing what's right for you. The answers to these questions quite simply cannot be accessed through our normal decision-making processes. What is required is an alternate option: the option of letting go in order to make the space to receive meaningful guidance from the depths of our own divinely inspired intuition.

There's a wonderful story from the Indian tradition that illustrates this option. A young disciple travels all the way across the country to seek out a certain spiritual master, renowned for his wisdom. When he finally arrives at his door, the master readily invites him in.

"Honored teacher, please share with me the answers to the questions I have been seeking." The student then goes on to impress the teacher with his qualifications for disciplehood: the earnestness of his spiritual preparation, the arduous nature of his journey.

The master responds, "I will do what you ask, but first join me for a cup of tea."

The master and the student sit down at the table, the student bubbling over with commentary about his hard work and self-discipline. As he talks, the master begins pouring the tea from the pot into the student's cup. The cup gets fuller and fuller until finally, it begins to overflow the top, onto the table and into his lap.

"Master!" the student exclaims. "You're spilling the tea!"

The master smiles.

"You are like this cup of tea! So full, there's room for no more. Come to me empty, then we can begin."

Interestingly enough, the patients who bury themselves at the medical library looking for answers and the patients who decide to let their doctors call all the shots all come to the decision-making process with full cups. As the master taught, what is required of us, particularly at critical junctures of our lives, is a letting go on the deepest levels. We cannot always rely on our own will and drive to bring us answers to the deeper questions. Nor can we relinquish our responsibility for answering these questions by asking others to decide for us. The third option is to empty our cups, making room for answers to well up in us from a deeper source, a source beyond our rational control.

This may sound esoteric. But we've all had experiences with this deeper kind of knowing. For instance, have you ever lost your car keys? What did you do? If you are like most people, you go back and search every possible place you can remember. Where were you the last time you saw the keys? What coat were you wearing? Who were you with?

These kinds of questions are the logical place to begin. Often, you find your keys. Of course, if you can solve your problems using the logical approach, you should do so. But what about those times you have gone through your entire bag of tricks, and still no keys? What do you do then? Chances are you give up. You say, "I'll go wash the dishes," or you go to read a book. And then what happens? The moment you put your attention elsewhere, the location of the keys pops into your mind. Did you make the answer happen? No. What you did was make space for it to come to you. We can't make our deeper answers happen. The best we can do is create the environment in which resolution is most likely to take place.

Over the years, I've developed numerous techniques that help me become receptive to possibilities outside of my rational control. I journal, I think about my dreams, I meditate, I pray. But most of all, I take long walks. So it was that when my doctor presented me with the possibility of joining a clinical trial, I took the time he offered to decide what to do. The study I was invited to join held the promise of greatly reducing my chances for a recurrence of breast cancer. There was one hitch. Those of us who chose to participate in the trial were submitting our bodies to the largest dosages of a particular combination of poisonous chemicals than had ever been tried before. The doctor explained that the trial had been going on for some time and that those who came before me were doing very well as a group. But even so, by participating in this trial, my regimen of chemotherapy and the attendant risks would be much greater than what I would otherwise undergo.

What should I do? I had no idea. I called my brother, a physician on the West Coast, to talk it over with him. He looked it over and said it looked acceptable to him, but that it was truly my decision. I talked to Dan and my friends. I made lists balancing and weighing the options. I looked for advice on the Internet. And when I still had no idea what to do, I decided to take the decision for a walk at Radnor Lake, the cousin to Walden Pond that is blessedly just one block from my house.

The last time I had been to Radnor Lake, I was with my daughter Jody. It was before my diagnosis and now seemed a long, long time ago. As we walked together down the shady paths, lined with bushes and trees, Jody had noticed something round and green in the underbrush.

She picked it up and showed it to me. It was a baby turtle—the kind you used to be able to buy in pet stores. I was overcome with excitement. As a young child, Jody's age, I'd had a turtle just like this one. I'd kept it in a plastic turtle bowl that had come complete with a miniature brown and green palm tree. In fact, I still had the turtle bowl somewhere in the attic. I had always wanted Jody to have a turtle like the one I'd had—and here it was, in the palm of her hand. I was certain that this turtle was the universe's gift to us and that we were meant to take it home with us and care for it.

I could see that Jody wanted this turtle more than anything in the world. She carried it with her partway around the trail, delighted as its little wiggling feet tickled her palm. But something was bothering her.

"It doesn't feel right to me, Mom," she said at last. "I think we've got to let it go."

To tell you the truth, I had the same feeling deep in the pit of my stomach. When we put the little turtle back into the underbrush, I felt like I was letting go my last chance for a childhood dream. I was so sad. But it was the right thing to do.

Now several months later, I was back at Radnor Lake, alone this time. The loss of the turtle was but the first of many losses I had suffered since my last visit. The loss of my breast. The loss of my self-image as a healthy woman. Now I was faced with making a decision that had to do with the possible loss of my life. In the parking lot, I prayed that by the time I completed the hourlong circle around the lake, I would know what to do about the clinical trial. And then I put it as far from my mind as I could, and started down the path. At first, it was an effort not to worry and think. But after a half-hour or so, I was finally able to take in the beauty around me, forgetting about my serious task. I heard a goose honk in the distance. Shiny green flies buzzed around my feet. I followed the path as it wound lazily around a corner. And there, standing silently, directly in the middle of the path—facing straight toward me—was the biggest turtle I had ever seen at Radnor Lake. It was at least two feet across. The creature fixed its wise eyes on mine and we communicated. It wasn't words. It wasn't even feelings. I just suddenly knew.

This was the baby turtle's mother. She was grateful to me for releasing her child. And what's more, I had been asking myself the wrong question about the clinical trial. It was not about whether I would live or die. It was about what I could do for the next generation. Live or die, because of me, if I were to participate in the trial, my daughter's generation would have better options for the treatment of breast cancer. My life would have been about something greater than myself.

We stood eye to eye for many moments, and then the turtle slowly, deliberately lumbered back up the path and disappeared into the brush. I stood there weeping in gratitude. I knew without any doubt that I was going to take the risk of participating in the trial, no matter what the cost might be to me personally.

What I have learned over this past year is that when it comes to making decisions, the most important thing I can do is to surrender my will, allowing myself to become receptive to forces greater than myself. Everything else is details. This is tougher than it may sound, since it entails the willingness to take the risk of believing in a loving and merciful God. Albert Einstein once said that the biggest question every individual must ask of himself or herself is this: whether this is a loving and orderly universe—or not.

Trust that there are forces working on your behalf every moment of your life. Quiet yourself and you will spontaneously relax into alignment with the unseen order of the universe. Look at yourself and your challenges through God's eyes and allow yourself to be empty enough to receive.

Here is a prayer from the Reform Judaism Sabbath service:

"O God, when doubt troubles us, when anxiety makes us tremble, and pain clouds the mind, we look inward for the answer to our prayers. There may we find you, and there find courage, insight, and endurance."

Amen.

Susan

Perhaps it is my age, my temperament, or my spiritual practice, but try as I may, I cannot answer the question, "Does God get to vote?" It seems the same as "Why do bad things happen to good people?" When terrible things happen to me, I am more interested in discovering the purpose than dwelling on the cause. I ask the question, "Why did this happen?" only if there is something I can do to prevent it in the future. For things that seem beyond my control, like breast cancer, I ask, "What can I learn?" If I had to picture God as anything, it would not be someone who votes, but a wild teacher, creating outlandish curricula to stretch my knowledge. Cancer may be one of the more advanced courses. So where can I find a study guide?

Carol's book *Solved by Sunset* is a guide to considering impossible questions. The method asks us to recognize and name an entire cast of inner voices. In the course of a one-day retreat, the voices are given a chance to speak. When I think about the question "Does God get to vote?" these are the voices that appear.

The first voice is the Dervish, the part of myself that is described in the metaphor of the Sufi poets as a "Drunkard in the Tavern of Ruin." Things may be falling down around me, but I revel in the disaster, knowing that as the outer world disintegrates, the inner world comes clearly into view. I am intoxicated with the wine of divine love.

My second voice is the Sufferer. I feel captured and weighted down by my own suffering and the suffering of others. It is beyond my comprehension. It feels as if it will never end.

My third voice is the Puzzled one. Why is it that there are so many more questions than answers? What does it all mean? The Sufis say that even God is puzzled.

My next voice is the Thinker. I like to study, to analyze situations, to think, and to learn. I was a philosophy major in college. For years, I had silenced this voice of the intellect, feeling it had no place on the spiritual path. That was a mistake. Intellectual inquiry is the perfect balance to devotion. All the great religious traditions have had thinkers, testing and refining the rules.

Finally, there is the voice I call the Knower. Perhaps it is too grand a word for this voice. This voice comes from the deepest part of my being, that which includes all of me yet seems to reach beyond me, into truth, or spirit, or what some might call God.

Here is the discussion among those inner voices:

Dervish: Does God get to vote? What an absurd question. Our concept of God stands in the way of our knowledge of God. Forget these questions. Come and join me as I dance and sing on the burial ground. My body is a cloak. My home is the soul.

Sufferer: I am praying to God. I want to get well. I am not ready to die. I am afraid.

Puzzled: How does God vote anyway? This isn't the suffering question, is it? Not the suffering question. Anything but the suffering question. It makes me crazy.

Thinker: The theologians grapple with this question. If God is good and compassionate, then why is there so much suffering? Buddha dealt with this suffering, as did Christ. There are many answers, but ultimately, this question is answered more from faith than from the intellect. Suffering is part of life's fullness; it coexists with an abiding trust in God's compassion and love.

Sufferer: The doctors and nurses notice that the nicest people get the worst diseases. I may die from my disease. I may die alone and in great pain. Does God choose this for me? Is this how God votes?

Knower: I have moments when I know. What is it that I know? I cannot say. A deep sense of knowing comes over me, something that I cannot put into words. I am blessed when I am in this state, and bereft when it is gone. But I can remember it. This sense of knowing is more real than objects or thoughts.

It is not my faith that brings this knowing, or my effort. It feels like an opening to a sense of rightness that is beyond suffering or salvation. It simply is. This knowing has come with my illness, I am certain. It hides like a secret. And who is the keeper of this secret? This is the God who attracts me, not the God who votes, or the God who is all-powerful, or the God who punishes, or the God who heals. This God is the secret of my heart.

As my voices grappled with the question, they led me to a sense of inner knowing. I was familiar with this place from my daily meditation practice. If meditation can be described in a sentence, it is listening to the inner voice of the heart. My diagnosis unnerved me. The fears and agitation made me forget about this place of knowing, this haven, this sanctuary. I was not ready to have cancer. I was too young. Too busy. Too alive.

I do not understand why or how our particular tragedies are dispensed, whether or not God votes. Yet, in the midst of the chaos, I rediscovered the secret knowing, quiet and hidden. I cannot name it. I cannot summon it when I need it most. But I can remember. It is the answer to every question, the answer that comes from spirit instead of logic. Others with cancer have told me that they have had a moment, an inkling of this inner knowing. There is no need to wait for the onset of disease to find this place. The way is always open.

Linda

One of the greatest blessings of my life is that no one in the circle of people who love me has ever threatened me with God's vengeance. So just as I believed that I did not cause my cancer, neither did I believe that God caused it—or that God somehow wanted me to have it.

I also believed that neither of us would take it away.

We shared the experience, God and I. We walked through the valley of the shadow of death. Goodness and mercy followed us, even though there were hills to climb that I had never imagined, and, on occasion, descents into depths also unimaginable.

But it was a partnership, a bipartisan effort of two of us who had elected to make this pilgrimage. There was no vote that either of us made regarding whether or not to go on this journey. It just was. And is.

I had to believe that there was a reason for the journey, I had to believe that I was moving forward with God's help and support, and toward his ultimate gift of peace.

Admittedly, it has been difficult to face life-threatening illness. But my therapist reminded me that "the same fire that melts the butter forges the steel." There is strength to be had from adversity—cancer counts—and greater peace to be had just beyond last hill.

That peace, and its gifts, is what I think that God, however we think of him (or her), wants for all of us. If God votes, he votes "Yes"—yes to the journey, yes to the learning, yes to my life, to your life, for whatever days there are to be.

Karen

I am ashamed to say that God had very little part in any of the decisions I made about my cancer treatment. On the other hand, she will get the important vote on the major, central issue. But first, history.

I went to the Vanderbilt Breast Center for my mammogram, needle biopsy, and surgery because I was a Vanderbilt student, and campus Student Health naturally referred everyone to Vanderbilt. My surgeon suggested a lumpectomy rather than a mastectomy and I was all too ready to agree, for what I now see are not very good reasons: I wanted to believe that this cancer was going to have a minimal impact on my life, and a lumpectomy fit in with that scenario better than did a mastectomy. Women's magazines have been touting the superiority of lumpectomies for years. I was engaged, and was afraid a mastectomy would send my fiancé screaming off into the night. And I was vain. This decision worked out all right in one way: I have had no trouble at the site of the original tumor. On the other hand, I am so small-breasted and the tumor was so large that some of my medical records refer to my surgery as a "partial mastectomy." But it never occurred to me to ask God what her desires in the matter were.

The surgeon's office made appointments for me to go to the radiation and medical oncologists. I had no decisions to make about radiation. I had one to make about chemotherapy: CMF or CAF? The second was "more difficult" to take, I was told, but would give me a 1 or 2 percent better chance at survival. I asked the doctor, "If I were your wife, what would you recommend?" He said CAF, and so I endured the dreaded adriamycin. I didn't "lift up" CMF versus CAF to God at all.

When I found out that my cancer had metastasized, I was offered a clinical trial. It was then I thought about going to M. D. Anderson, the premier cancer center in this country. But since I was a poor graduate student who had not worked in six months, that was out of the question. My doctor suggested the clinical trial gave me the best chance for survival, so I signed the papers right then. Even if I had thought to give God a vote in this matter, practical considerations made it a futile exercise.

When it turned out the trial was not working, again I was offered one option: ninety-six-hour infusions of Taxol every four weeks. Again I immediately made an appointment for treatment starting the following Monday.

Through all of this, my relationship with God was definitely alive. I knew I got through the horrors of treatment only because God was sustaining me. I kept hope because I knew so many people were praying for me and I thought that might convince God to let me live a while longer. But I did not ask God what she wanted. I did not give her a vote. Instead, I gave her what was almost a command. When I prayed, I said, again and again, "I want to live." When I saw a cardinal on the wing, I said, "I want to live." When I saw a shooting star, I said, "I want to live." And as I soothed myself to sleep, I used this mantra: "I want to live. I want to live. I want to live."

And so I did. As I said, I am ashamed that it never occurred to me to ask, "What direction does God want me to take in my treatment?" Me, the Christian minister. This is even more ironic because I am trained as an Ignatian spiritual director, and part of that tradition is learning to "discern the spirits," learning to figure out what God wants in a situation. But it was almost as if I were afraid to find out—there was always the possibility that God was ready for me to die, and I simply could not entertain the thought.

On the other hand, my spiritual director reminded me of something I know but often need to be reminded of: God wants life, not death. I had no idea before the cancer how strong the will to live was in me. I had no idea that I could go through so much and still want to be around. I did not think I had that much stamina. People have often said to me, "Oh, you're such an inspiration," but I have always rejected that, because from my point of view, I was simply doing what I had to do to obey that primitive voice coming from deep inside of me: *I want to live.* I am tempted to say that God's vote came in the "still, small voice," but there was nothing still or small about that voice.

But perhaps I was saving God's vote for the big decision. That makes no sense, of course. It is not as if I get a quota of God's attention and am in danger of running through it like a new lottery winner goes through prize money. But cancer is not logical. Anyway, the fact is that sooner or later this treatment I am on will stop working. It has been a wonderful treatment; I take pills twice a day and have an implant once a month. I have no side effects except hot flashes and no menstrual cycles. But it will not last forever. I have—perhaps foolishly—read too many medical articles and know that the average length of time this drug works before the cancer builds up a resistance to it is two years. So far, I have beaten the average by six months. I hope to beat it by a lot more, but I also try to stay realistic. And when the time comes, I will have a major decision to make: Do I try more chemotherapy, or do I just enjoy my last six months and go?

A woman in my support group had ovarian cancer and heard the dreaded news from the doctor that "there's nothing more we can do." So she gathered her friends together and asked them to help her make a decision—stop trying to find a treatment, search like mad for something experimental, or try alternative therapies. As a group, they helped her decide on the third option. And she died just when the doctors said she would.

When my cancer starts growing again, there will, I have no doubt, be a part of me that chants, "I want to live, I want to live, I want to live" as it always has. Part of me will want to live no matter what living is like. That part cannot consider quality versus quantity. But then there is another part of me, the part that knows what it is like to live with unending chemo, and cannot imagine having chemo up until the day I die. That is the part of me that finds dying scary but knows death promises something better than this world. That is also the part of me that realizes the work I have to do here in this life is probably complete. I have no husband, no children to love and nurture. I have good and important work, but it is work that many others could do. So at that point, the question will be, "Do I keep on trying to stay alive, or go gently into that dark night?"

God gets to answer that question, and I am ready for whatever the answer might be. As odd as it might sound, I can stand the idea of death better now than I could when I was in the middle of the misery of treatment. Perhaps it has just taken a long time for God to work in me so I am more open to both possibilities. A priest who works at Lourdes says the people who get miraculous cures are *not* the ones who simply *have* to have them, but those who are at peace with whatever God decides to send into their lives. I cannot say I am perfectly at peace with the prospect of dying, but I am a lot closer than I was just a few years ago.

I will pray about this decision, certainly, but I will also borrow from my friends in support group. I will gather together the people in my life: friends, relatives, people who have ministered to me, therapists, doctors, and nurses. We will have a simple worship service that starts with prayers for wisdom and discernment and goes on to offer several Scripture passages about trusting in God. The "sermon" will be a group effort. People will go off by themselves for a while to pray, then come back together and talk. I plan to have an active part in this discussion, but I also believe strongly that we learn God's will partly through community. If it is the sense of the community for which God wants me to continue the struggle to live, I will do so—counting on all those people to help me bear the treatment, and leaning on their hope for me when I cannot hope for myself. And if the community senses it is time for me to go, I will do so. I will need to count on those people even more in that situation.

But maybe not. Maybe the voice that says "I want to live" *is* God's vote. I cannot answer that question right now; just as was the case when I was first diagnosed, I cannot know in advance how I will react. My prayer these days is that it will be a long time before the voting begins.

Choices

THERE IS LITTLE TIME TO LINGER IN CHAOS. Treatment choices must be examined and decisions made. Is treatment war or initiation? Do I hold on or do I let go? Do I trust the medical establishment or do I put my faith in alternative and spiritual healing resources? We must educate ourselves rapidly on what choices are available, decide what to do, and do it. Since the cure for cancer is not known, there is much uncertainty. Options are presented in terms of percentages.

The underlying issue is learning to trust. There are many alternatives and no one "right" way. Being spiritual does not exclude medical science and vice versa.

Others can support your treatment choices. They can listen to you, enter your view of your situation, and speak with you from this perspective.

You gain strength, courage, and confidence by every
experience in which you really stop to look fear
in the face. You must do the thing which
you think you cannot do.
—ELEANOR ROOSEVELT

In the prevailing terminology, treatment is the battle-ground upon which a war against cancer is fought. We women routinely tough it out, continuing to work, take care of our families and the like, determined to show that we are bigger and stronger than our disease. As a result, we are often burned out and spiritually deprived by what could be one of the richest and deepest experiences of our lives.

The spiritual approach to breast cancer treatment views the pain and challenge as initiation, not war. Treatment, when viewed through a spiritual lens, can be seen as sanctification, purification, and even sacrifice. Spiritual tools and resources may be called upon to turn treatment, painful as it may be, into initiation.

The choices are not always, perhaps never, easy. Even women with well-developed religious lives can fall into spiritual pitfalls when faced with their own mortality. The question often posed is whether the best spiritual stance is to fight for one's life, whether through traditional medicine or alternative treatment or some combination of the two, or to surrender to God's will and/or divine destiny. This is a question that leads many women into unnecessary pain. Perhaps the real answer lies in a more evolved understanding of the meaning of acceptance: How is it possible both to do everything you can within your power to live your life to the fullest, and put your destiny in God's hands?

FOUR

Is Treatment War
or Initiation?

Linda

War is hell.

So, no, I don't think I'll enlist.

Granted, the diagnosis of a life-threatening illness is tantamount to a draft notice, and to keep from joining the fight, you will probably need to reject some established medical thinking. My experience, however, convinced me that early surrender could save my spirit, if not my life. It seemed to me that was quite a deal.

For me, treatment began with surgery, followed by six months of chemotherapy, then seven weeks of radiation.

Was it a battle plan? Did it establish a line of defense? Would it be a fight to the finish?

No.

It was a rite of passage, moving into the next phase of a journey that would take me toward wholeness—minus a breast, but whole nevertheless.

When I began chemotherapy, an unusually long time after my mastectomy because of post-op complications, I was mentally and emotionally prepared.

If you'd seen me that day, however, you might not have guessed it, since I dressed for my first treatment wearing a T-shirt bearing skulls and other bony symbols of Mexico's Day of the Dead.

It seemed to be a way to say that no matter what the outcome, there will be cause to celebrate. Once treatment began, sometimes it was harder to remember that.

And, for me, there was extra time to think about it, even after I had decided that I would follow the recommended course of chemotherapy, after they had told me what to expect.

That's because a little more than a week after my initial surgery, I was told that I was "losing tissue" in the reconstructed breast—a portion of the tissue that had been replanted from my abdomen to my chest was "not taking."

It happens, although not often. But when it happens to you, you don't really care that it didn't happen to 1,000 previous patients and it won't happen to the next 1,000.

The incision was reopened, and the plastic surgeon removed dead tissue—abdominal tissue that obviously had decided it did not want to become a breast.

I went home with a gaping wound because the incision had to remain open.

At this point, you must remember that I am a journalist, not a nurse or a doctor or an EMT. I write feature stories for a newspaper, and it's been years since I covered a bloody news event.

For twelve weeks my bathroom became a field hospital. Twice a day I had to slip off the stretchy mesh "tube top" that held all the bandages in place, don disposable latex gloves, and remove layers of gauze until I exposed this vast hole in my chest. Seriously, it was open about eight inches, from the middle of what used to be my breast back to my armpit, and it was a couple of inches deep. I could look in it—I could see inside my body, like the plastic Visible Woman I got for Christmas when I was in the fifth grade.

What we—I had become part of the medical team—had to do was something called "debridement," removing tissue as it died so that the path was clear for healthy new tissue to grow.

I would shower and let the water wash away whatever portion of the dying tissue that was ready to detach, then pour Dakin solution—the pharmaceutical name for diluted household bleach—into the wound. Then I had to pack the whole thing with about a dozen yards of gauze (no, I am not exaggerating), put an antiseptic cream on just the edges of the wound, and then cover it all up again.

It was not pretty.

When I first had to do wound care, I hated it. I'd shower in the dark, so the only time I'd really have to look at the bloody tissue was when I dressed it again.

After a week, it became routine, as so many things would over the next eight months. Perhaps I had been initiated after all, perhaps I was a member of a club that, like Gilda Radner once said, nobody really wants to be a member of.

So, I accepted it. I put one foot in front of the other (and one gloved hand in my chest), but when there was enough healthy tissue to allow the doctor to close the wound, I was thrilled. The thrill was short-lived, however.

A few days later, I developed a massive infection that refused to respond to oral antibiotics. The wound had to be reopened. I thought it was the worst thing that would happen; it wasn't.

I returned to the hospital for a week of intravenous antibiotics. By then I was seriously into looking at the bright side whenever I could—and the bright side was that at the hospital the nurses changed the dressing. I couldn't have been happier—well, I could've, but under the circumstances, that was as good as it was going to get.

In fact, it was going to get much worse. Chemotherapy introduces into your system drugs that are toxic to the cancer cells, and they chase them and kill them. Of course, the drugs don't know the difference between a cancer cell and a healthy cell, so they attack every fast-growing cell in their path. Needless to say, the process plays hell with your immune system.

The start of chemotherapy was delayed because I had an open wound and didn't want to risk further infection (nor did I want to prolong my newfound nursing career). It was almost two months after surgery before I could begin chemotherapy, and another month before they completely closed the chest wound.

I had heard the chemo stories and was dreading it, but, hey, how bad could it be? After all, hadn't I gone through the initiation already?

The treatment regimen that the medical oncologist had chosen for me was something called CAF—a combination of three drugs, Cytoxan, adriamycin, and 5-fluorouracil. I'd have a treatment on two consecutive Fridays, then skip two, until I'd finished six rounds.

The time each treatment takes varies, depending on the drugs. Mine took about two hours each time, lying back in the medical version of a La-Z-Boy while they drip about $1,000 worth of toxins into your veins.

Fortunately, those who poisoned me to make me well were terrific people. They understood my fears, and they never, ever tried to minimize what was happening to me. I was hooked up to an IV, and an antinausea drug, Zofran, was started. After a few minutes, it was time to start the drugs that were going to (a) attack the cancer cells and (b) make me very sick. "One out of two's not bad," I thought.

"We call this the red devil," the nurse said as she sat down beside me with a huge syringe that looked like it was filled with strawberry Jell-O. That was the adriamycin, the drug they promised would cause my hair to fall out in two weeks flat. I counted it a major victory when I made it seventeen days.

The adriamycin was administered by a "push," that is, the nurse held the syringe that she'd fastened to the needle that was in my arm and eased the thick, red chemotherapy drug into my vein. When that was done, one more drug was pushed, then the remainder that were in bags hanging from the IV pole like some bizarre jellyfish were then allowed to drip through the tubing and into my arm.

When we were done, the nurse reminded me that adriamycin is particularly toxic, so they don't want it to sit in your bladder. "Drink plenty of water and pee like a racehorse," she said. Jeez, I thought, something else to look forward to.

But before I could be a full-fledged member of the club of people bound by cancer treatment, I would be called on for another sacrifice. First, it was my breast. Next, my hair. I have very thick hair, so I was able to hold on to my denial about hair loss for a while. After the second round of chemo, a week after the first, I began counting the days. On the morning of the tenth day, my pillow was, well, hairy. Clumps of hair were stuck to my face. Ditto the morning of the eleventh day. So I washed and dried my hair very gently—like it was gonna help, huh?— and decided it was certainly thinner, but there were no major bald spots.

I went to work. At noon I was sitting at my desk typing when this big chunk of hair fell onto my keyboard. I quickly looked around to see if anybody had seen it, sort of like if you're walking into church and your slip falls down. Then I went home and cried.

I'd already lost a breast, so in the greater scheme of things, hair shouldn't be a big deal. (And hair does come back.) But it's such a visible loss, an ever-present reminder that your life is very different.

The next day, I wore a hat and scarf to work, a black gaucho number that was rather stylish, but I still felt like I was in my freshman beanie, letting people know that I was an initiate and once hell week was over (even though it might last for years), I'd be just like everyone else. Right.

Every day for the next eight months, except for those days late in treatment when I could hardly lift my head, much less put a hat on it, I wore a scarf or bandana and a hat or a baseball cap.

After the initial hair loss, a few patches remained. When I was a kid, my mother always told me never to put my head on the back of the seat in the movie; if I did, I'd get ringworm. Now I knew what I would've looked like if I had not obeyed her. I thought it would be an improvement to have my head shaved, so my hairdresser obliged. OK, that's done, I thought. But what nobody tells you—maybe they think you know—is that you lose all your body hair. One day you realize you haven't shaved your legs in weeks and they're silky smooth. And that downy fuzz on your face that gets annoyingly more obvious in middle age? Gone. I was, as we say in the South, "nekkid as a jaybird." I was astounded at how very, very vulnerable I felt.

The first two times chemotherapy was administered, my veins rebelled. If the nurse managed to get "a good stick," it wouldn't hold up for the two-hour duration of the treatment. That meant another stick, and usually another. It was not a promising beginning for the remaining months of treatment. The solution was a "port," a stainless steel catheter implanted just beneath my collarbone to provide ready access to the subclavian vein running below it.

All the while, I was trying to keep myself emotionally steady, but I felt like I was being fitted out for battle. It was hard to stay focused with a flurry of activity surrounding me on every treatment day. The images, the descriptions of cancer treatment were more violent than I had hoped—I had never been aware before that so many people were "fighting" cancer, "battling" their disease, "struggling to survive," "coming face to face with the enemy."

Not me, I said. I'm a conscientious objector and I won't go to war with you. But, hey, I'm always up for a picnic. Just let me get my hat.

Carol

Toward the end of chemotherapy, I began to think about the future. I had received an invitation to lead a seminar in Munich in conjunction with the publication of *The Art of Resilience* in German. On one of my many visits to the cancer clinic, I asked my oncologist his advice. Should I go?

Always attentive and helpful,—without stepping over the line of telling me what I should or had to do—my doctor told me his own story. He himself had been diagnosed and treated for cancer not long ago. And near the end of his chemotherapy, he too received an invitation to go to Europe to deliver an important paper.

"Did you accept?" I asked.

"Sure did. I basically unplugged the tubing and got on a flight to Denmark."

I thought hopefully about his remark for the several weeks between appointments. But as I gauged my own energy level, I began to doubt that I would have the stamina to carry on as he had. The next visit, I brought up the subject again.

"Doctor, you told me you got on a plane to go to Europe, but you didn't tell me how it turned out! How did it go?"

Without a moment's hesitation, he heartily responded: "Terrible. It was a big mistake!"

It turns out that upon arrival in Europe, his mouth, hands, and feet had a serious delayed reaction. They became so sore and tender, he was not able to hold his own fork or walk across the floor. Face to face with an array of European pastries the likes of which he had never seen before, he could neither swallow nor chew. I suggested that perhaps I postpone the trip for a year. All who heard the story, including the nurses who hovered nearby, nodded relieved assent.

Stories about the victory of the human spirit over cancer inspire others. But I wonder if the inspiration comes more often than not at the heroine's own expense? Common sense—and the more holistic approach to body-mind-spirit that I'd been following since the '60s—would suggest that when your body is ill, you need rest. I'm not talking about becoming a couch potato, giving up and going into hiding. But I am suggesting that we all need balance in our lives: times when we are driving ourselves through the force of will, and times when we are nurturing ourselves by letting go and relaxing deeply. This is true for all of us, and doubly true for people dealing with serious illness. Cancer cells are parts of our own bodies that don't recognize their own boundaries and limitations. Ironically, the cancer culture honors exactly those traits that may have contributed to our immune system's exhaustion in the first place: raging, racing, and fighting to win.

From the beginning, I related to my cancer differently. I was an antiwar activist in the '60s: a member of the "make love, not war" generation. I refused to wage war against my own body—even part of me that had gone awry. Surely there was some other metaphor that could be both inspirational and life giving.

I found my metaphor in my journals, the daily record of my spiritual journey. For years, I had been learning to surrender control and to have faith in myself and in God. Could my breast cancer be a spiritual initiation into deeper levels of understanding and experience, and not a battle to be waged against the enemy? In one of my first meditations after diagnosis, it came to me that it was no accident that it was my left breast that carried the illness. My left breast: the breast nearest to my heart (as the majority of women's breast cancers are). Year after year, I had made the attempt to absorb the cruelty, stupidity, and fear that I encountered in the course of running my business, career, and life, vowing to do everything in my power not to pass it on. I had prevailed upon my heart to process the negativity, making the effort to transform it into the light of compassion and understanding. Sometimes I succeeded, sometimes I did not. In my vision, I saw my left breast as a filter, cleansing the debris of life on its way to my vulnerable heart. At last, my heart had grown strong enough to handle life's challenges without the layers of protection. With the doctor's announcement that I was going to need a mastectomy, I realized that my left breast's job was complete. Letting it go was to be my personal sacrifice.

The night before the operation, I gathered my family around the fireplace in the living room. I had a ritual I wanted to share with them. I surrendered to the loss of my breast, but I wanted it to be for some higher meaning. So I asked each of them to think of something in their life that had already fulfilled its purpose—an outmoded belief or behavior that they no longer wanted or needed—to write it down on a piece of paper and throw it into the fire. As we watched the papers go up in flames, I asked God that along with my breast, these old beliefs and behaviors be released. If I needed any more confirmation that this ritual sacrifice had been inspired by God, I got it on the pre-op table immediately before surgery. Just before closing my eyes, I noticed the nametag of my anesthesiologist. The doctor's name was Pascal: the Biblical reference to the sacrificial lamb.

At this point in my journey through life, allowing myself to be vulnerable, even if the wounding carries pain with it, is a better way for me to be in the world. There are aching cracks in my facade that weren't there before. Unlike survivors who have battled their cancer to emerge victoriously unchanged, I have been cracked open to the very core of my being. But it is through these cracks, in the fertile ground of my vulnerable heart, that the tender sprouts of music, poetry, love, and friendship have taken root.

By the time I began chemotherapy, I was already melted and defenseless. But I was not a victim. Even though I had surrendered the illusion of my personal power, there was something powerful going on in my life.

This sense of empowerment included my decision to take part in the clinical trial, allowing myself to be used as a human guinea pig to benefit those who would come after me. It turned out that those of us who volunteered for the study were to be divided into two groups. One group was to get six treatments, the other seven. The group I would be assigned to was determined by chance. Nobody in their right mind would hope to get the larger number of rounds. But I did. Seven is the day of the week associated with the Jewish Sabbath—the day of rest that completes the cycle of the seven days of creation. In Eastern mysticism, seven is also the number of completion. When my nurse broke the news to me, apologizing for the added round, I told her that I was prepared for the seven courses of treatment. I anticipated the treatment as cleansing and purifying, the completion of the job the sacrifice of my breast had begun. I knew from my spiritual and psychological studies as a graduate student that new habits take time to set. I wanted to use this time to elevate myself to a higher plane. The seven rounds felt just right to me.

I surrendered to my seven rounds of chemotherapy, but I was still scared. God was kind, and gave me a chemo nurse who held my hand through the whole experience. Even though she walked into my treatment cubicle a stranger to me, I saw from the very first in her seasoned eyes a depth of love and compassion I longed to emulate in my own life. My nurse midwifed the dissolution of my false bravado and the birth of something new and tender in my spirit. I learned by receiving, a new way of being for me.

When I gazed up in terror at the red liquid that was to be pumped into my heart, she convinced me to think of it not as poison, but as medicine, working with me on the deepest levels to cleanse and purify my body and spirit. Before she turned the intravenous machinery on, she made sure I was warm and comfortable, bringing me a blanket and turning down the light. I put on my earphones, trying to calm myself down enough to tune into the tape of rhythmic spiritual chants I had selected. She sat with me until I was ready and then, at last, she flipped open the switch. I watched silently as the red liquid began its methodical journey down the tubing and into my heart, one drop at a time. The drops came in a steady beat: drip drip drip. There was a rhythm to the drops. I watched in fascination. What was it about the drops that after all the fearful anticipation felt so deeply comforting to me? And then suddenly, I realized what it was. Miraculously, the drops were descending in the exact rhythm as the chanting in my earphones. There was a synchronicity, a unity to the initiation of my chemotherapy that was beyond accidental. I was healing myself of cancer, not as a soldier, but as an initiate.

Susan

When you have breast cancer, frightening, high-stakes choices translate into life or death. The decisions come rapidly with no preparation, during a state of emotional shock. Few people understand how these choices are made, and how to support those of us who must make them. We give our permission by signing a document called informed consent, the "process," as Dr. Susan Love says in her book, "in which the patient is fully informed of all risks and complications of a planned procedure and agrees to proceed." It is an enlightened process, created to prevent experimentation on human subjects without informing them of the risks.

Informed consent is a foundation of ethical medical practice. Yet, it contains an inherent problem. How can a person be truly informed about the unknown? The longer I live with cancer, the more familiar I become with the precipice of the unknown. Like a mountain climber, I am prepared for high risk. Isn't life high risk? I had forgotten. I was lulled into comfort through consistent good health. Then, the terror. It crystallized on the day I had to sign the consent for my mastectomy. Like post-traumatic stress syndrome, I recall each detail.

I sat alone in the examining room of the clinic. The latest surgical resident came in with a blue triplicate form. He asked me if I had any questions about my surgery. Suddenly I understood. This was informed consent. He was required to ask me if I had any questions, a follow-up to the explanation of the "procedure" I had just heard from the surgeon, before he left the room to attend to his next patient. The young resident was a little nervous, as if he were trying to make a big sale. He volunteered no information. He had seen many surgeries. Surely there were some things he could tell me, but the professional curtain contained them.

I signed the form. Driving home after the appointment, I remembered with horror that I did not read what surgery I had signed for. My mind was in a tailspin.

How could I have asked my real questions? Will I die? Will the moments before my surgery be the last moments of my life? Should I say good-bye to the world and to those I love? I knew the resident would not answer these questions. He would quote the percentages. With the mastectomy I have a 3 to 5 percent chance of cancer recurring in that breast, usually at the scar. There is a 16 percent chance that I may get lymphedema, my arm bloated with fluid that my lymph system cannot drain. Radiation can cause that too. There is only a .2 percent chance of dying from anesthesia. Safer than driving to the hospital. I have a 90 percent chance of surviving tubular carcinoma. With lumpectomy and radiation I would have approximately a 10 percent chance of local recurrence in that breast. Whatever treatment, my life expectancy is about the same.

I was certain that I would die. On the morning of the surgery I had more questions. I asked my surgeon, "Can I walk into the operating room instead of being rolled in?" "No. You can sit up and crawl from the bed to the operating table." This was hardly my picture of dignity.

"Can you wait until I am in surgery to give me drugs?" I wanted to be awake as long as I could. He agreed to this. The nurse preparing me for the operation was surprised. Most people prefer the drugs.

I had another reason for being awake. I wanted to see the setting, the things of that world. How curious I am about all the stuff. I love the little, particular things of people's work that are so ordinary to them, so fascinating to me. I had so many questions that, at the time, I never asked. We had to stay focused on the business at hand.

How are all those blue pajamas stacked and labeled? Who designed those funny net helmets that the surgeons wear? They are so much more fashionable than the shower caps. Where will they put my breast? In one of those throw-up pans? Tupperware? How does it get to the pathologist?

What will it look like just lying there detached from me? Will it find me when the trumpets blow on Judgment Day and we all get to dance and sing once more?

What does it feel like to be a surgeon, to put your hands inside other people's bodies, then live with those hands all day? It is such a strange intimacy. How much practice will the residents get on me? What a test of trust. Does the operating room need a coat of paint? How do they clean up all the blood? Did people die in there? When? Are fragments of their souls hovering in the air? Where do they warm the blankets? Why is the operating room is so cold?

On the day I signed the consent form, did I look like a rational, educated woman? In a parallel universe, the vast unknown locked down the surface of my mind, completely isolated from the well of meaning. Underneath the sane, rational signing of the contract was my wild, elemental dialogue with death, the dark womb of the mother who gave me a body and was claiming it once again for herself.

The day came. Minutes before the operation, my surgeon stood at the foot of my rolling bed, checking the informed consent document. In one of the fill-in-the-blank lines, he had forgotten to specify which breast. He took a pen out of his pocket, and wrote in "left." My choice ended with that gesture. So did my breast.

Is treatment war or initiation? I did not feel like a warrior. I am naturally more curious than combative, more a student than a conqueror. I did not want to fight. I wanted to understand. I continue to read articles and attend lectures, as I try to master the known.

Medical science advances by delving into the unknown and, bit by bit, bringing new knowledge to the surface. In one of the real miracles of modern science, the medical community has an elegant system to collect, report, share, and apply this knowledge. So many of us are alive because of it.

The current knowledge about breast cancer is incomplete. Breast cancer treatment is a step into the unknown. That's why informed consent is a moment of initiation. The Sufi mystic Inayat Khan says, "Initiation is taking a step forward in a direction one does not know." Choosing to enter the unknown requires the greatest courage.

Understanding the unknowable is the realm of mystics and poets.

Like scientists and explorers, they chart this territory. They describe it with a language that reaches beyond words. In the *Sufi Message*, Inayat Khan goes on to say, "Sometimes initiation comes after great illness, pain, or suffering. It comes as an opening up of the horizon, and in a moment the world seems transformed. It is not that the world has changed, but that person is tuned to a different pitch. She begins to think, feel differently, and act differently, her whole condition begins to change. One might say that from that moment this person begins to live."

Cancer is but one way to step into the unknown. The initiate is poised to learn the language of faith and the science of the heart, to drown in unknowing and become transformed.

Karen

I just got off the telephone with a woman who has recently had what we all hope will be her last chemotherapy treatment for breast cancer. Her task now is to recover from treatment, get back to "normal" life, wait, and integrate what she has just been through. "I don't know who I am anymore," she said to me. "I mean, I'm still me, but it's a very different me."

I know exactly what she was talking about. Treatment for cancer is a life-changing experience. It has been over two years since I had chemotherapy, and I am still figuring out everything it meant.

I am, like my friend, still me, but very different. I find I have changed in ways that are not the same as other cancer patients I talk to, though. I hear tales from patients who used to put all their energy into work, and since treatment have paid more attention to their families. Others say they have become deeper people. But I cannot say either of these things. I think I had a pretty good balance in my life before cancer treatment, and quite honestly, I was a deep and compassionate person before all this. Still, I am changed, and in a radical way.

I bought into the military terminology for treatment at first. That is partly because that was all I had ever heard. I was a warrior, I told myself, fighting the cancer battle. I hoped to achieve victory on the battlefield and become a "survivor." I bought the video game "Doom" and visualized all the aliens I was killing as cancer cells. I read the psalms in which the speaker asks God to wreak vengeance on her enemies. For the first time in my life, I thought "Onward, Christian Soldiers" was an appropriate hymn. I found a picture of a breast cancer cell in a women's magazine and put it on a dart board. I was a warrior, no doubt about it. Or if not a soldier, then a boxer. I told a friend once, "I feel like I'm in a boxing ring, and I keep getting knocked down. I keep getting back up, but it's harder and harder every time."

But here is the reality: We are not "winning" the war on cancer, and we are not likely to do so anytime soon. Since President Nixon declared the war on cancer, countless wonder treatments that worked beautifully in laboratory animals have proven only partially beneficial to human beings. There have been some strides, of course. Hodgkin's disease is largely curable, as are testicular cancer and most childhood leukemias. But the cure rate for breast cancer has not changed since the beginning of this century. If this is a war, then it is not surprising that the troops are demoralized.

But I realized one day that such language was doing me no good. The fact is that my cancer is not cured, it is not technically in remission, and I have a terminal prognosis. So I have "lost the war." In the wartime vocabulary of cancer treatment, I am a loser. I have been defeated.

So why is it that I am a better person, a stronger person, a person who does not at all feel like a loser or a victim? I am a different person, but it is not because I have spent time as a soldier.

It came to me slowly that battle imagery would not work for me. But neither would visualizations of gentle waterfalls washing away my cancer cells; there was more agony in my life than waterfalls implied. I also could not manage to pull myself up by my bootstraps and simply decide to get well. I found my vocabulary, my way to speak about cancer treatment, in the world of faith, in the vocabulary of initiation. In particular, I rediscovered the ancient initiatory tale of the one who dies and rises again.

One of the stories that became very important to me during treatment is the myth of Inanna, a Sumerian goddess. The favorite offspring of her father, she gets him drunk and tricks him into giving her most of his powers. She is then a mighty force to be reckoned with, equally matched by her consort Dumuzi. But Inanna, strong as she is, has a trial to go through. She must travel to the underworld to see her sister, Ereshkigal. As Inanna goes deeper and deeper into the underworld, she is stripped. Off come her clothes, off come her powers, so that when she reaches Ereshkigal, Inanna is weakened and naked. Her sister greets her by killing her and hanging her body on a meat hook.

But Inanna comes back to life. She rises from the dead, still powerful but changed. Having been through the suffering she has endured, she is a different goddess.

Since I am the Christian voice in this book, it may seem strange that a pagan myth has been so important to me. After all, why not Jesus of Nazareth on the cross? That image has been critical for me, as well. But it is also true that as deeply as I allow myself to imagine the agony he went through, there is still a tiny little voice that speaks in the back of my head: "Yeah, but it was only six hours." Treatment, for me, lasted two and a half years. Inanna's journey better approximates my own.

But then again, who knows what Jesus went through in the three days he was dead? One gospel says he went down to hell to save the righteous, and three days in hell must have been a horror. And I imagine, too, that part of hell is that time is distorted. Who knows how long he suffered? I am definitely in the realm of speculation here, but as a Christian I yearn to find spiritual guidance in the history of my tradition.

So Jesus, like Inanna, rose from the dead. The difference between them is that Inanna was a mythic figure and Jesus a historical one. While myth may encompass Truth, there is something compelling about an actual human being going through these actual events. Jesus, then, led me to resurrection.

I have wondered if "being raised from the dead" is not a better metaphor than "resurrection." The story of Lazarus is probably more relevant to me than that of Jesus. The poor man had been dead and decomposing and Jesus raised him to life. Lazarus, though, had to face death again. That is more the situation I am in. And again, all I can do is speculate about how Lazarus spent the period between the time he was raised from the dead and his final death.

Finally, however helpful the stories of my faith and other myths are,

I am still left with my own experience. And my experience was that I went into hell and came back to life.

Taxol is a wonderful drug, as chemotherapies go. It is reasonably easy to take, and it does not cause the horrible nausea that so many medications do. But one of the side effects of Taxol is that people lose their hair. I lost my hair—every single strand on my head. And my face, and my armpits, and my legs, and my pubic area. I lost my eyebrows and the hair in my ears and my nose. When I could bear to look at myself naked in the mirror, what I saw was a newborn baby.

That physical manifestation was appropriate in many ways. I think of Reynolds Price, the wonderful writer who had a cancer that was finally cured but which left him in a wheelchair. He has written a book about his experience called *A Whole New Life.* I took a page from Price, and asked myself during treatment, "Who am I going to be now?"

I definitely had to be a new person. I could not remain the one who had never had cancer. For one thing, I now know what it is like to suffer deeply. Simply put, there are some people who understand that experience, and others who do not. By messing with my immune system, chemotherapy made my body more sensitive to allergens; I am now allergic to a thousand things.

In the same way, my soul became more sensitive to suffering. As I have already said, I was not a shallow or callous person before cancer. But now, having been through my initiation, I am always aware of the suffering that is going on in the world. That is most obvious to me in the congregation I pastor. These people are close to me, both emotionally and geographically, and so I know their suffering of all different kinds. I cannot have the same depth of knowledge about people on the other side of the world. But still, I am haunted by thoughts of starving children, brutalized women, and tortured men. It simply cannot be the case anymore that if things are well with me, then "all is right with the world." This awareness leaves my heart torn open almost all the time. That is painful, but I think it is the way Jesus probably lived.

In my descent into the depths, I have also become a different person in the way I view life. I know now how very, very precious it is. I know that each day a human being lives has some good in it, even if most of that day is misery. Even when I am having a terrible day—or a terrible year—I still want to live. I was and am surprised at how strong in me is the will to live. The fact that I endured my initiation does not speak to any level of bravery on my part. Instead, it simply says that I learned how much I want to live.

The other side of that coin is that while I love life now more than I ever thought possible, I hold it quite loosely these days. I know my cancer may start growing again tomorrow. I also know that I could die of a hundred causes this afternoon. And in an odd sort of way, that is all right. I have come to terms with the fact that I will die.

There is a long tradition in the Christian faith of people talking about suffering as a "refining fire." It made sense to me, then, when a friend in North Carolina wrote a song about me, with a line that says, "She sits hooked to a machine while the chemo cooks her veins." I have been burned, there is no doubt about it, and much was burned away. I think I am less judgmental than I was before. Or maybe not. I can see people's weaknesses and sinfulness so easily these days. Recognizing weakness and sin is a form of judgment. But what is different is that it does not make me feel any different about these people. If anything, I love them more not *in spite of* their foibles, but partly because of them.

Something else that got burned away was my concern about money. During treatment, I could not work, and so I worried about money all the time. But just when I got to the point that financial disaster loomed, money would appear from somewhere. Today I lead a very simple life; my salary will not allow me any other kind. But that is fine with me, and I do not worry about money any more. Somehow, I will get what I need.

Part of my initiation was sacrifice. Unlike many women, I did not sacrifice my whole breast. But the treatment I am on now takes all the estrogen out of my body. That means hot flashes and a lowered sex drive, but it also means one very important thing: I will never have a child. My plan when I entered graduate school was to get my degree, get a teaching job somewhere, and then have a baby whether I was married or not. That is simply impossible now. If the chemotherapy has not completely destroyed my ovaries, then the knowledge that the estrogen that comes with pregnancy would make my cancer grow keeps me from becoming pregnant. No adoption agency in the world is going to give a child to a single woman with a terminal prognosis. I love my nieces and nephew more than I ever thought possible, and I dote on the children in my congregation. Yet it is not the same as having a child of my own.

I think often about Jesus, and the fact that he apparently had no children. I wonder how much loss he felt about that fact, and whether he thought it a sacrifice. But again—he's a male savior, and I am just not certain he can understand how I feel. What makes sense to me is the neo-pagan idea of the three stages in a woman's life, which are the three faces of the goddess. The first is virgin, the second, mother, which are just what they say. But the third stage is the crone—the woman past childbearing age who has wisdom gleaned from life. I became a crone at thirty-six, which is a little early. And truth to tell, it is not that I was a young woman the day before I was diagnosed and a crone after my first chemotherapy treatment. Rather, it is an image I have grown into, and will continue to grow into.

Like the crone, I remind people of death. Even those who are reading these words may find it odd or distasteful that I talk about my cancer treatment as an initiation and yet obviously hated it so much. But that is the way real initiations are. We have lost that in our culture; the "initiations" we have now are silly and violent without purpose: sorority and fraternity initiations, military group initiations, secret societies. Real initiations involve pain, because one of the truths of the universe is that life is painful. But in a real initiation, the pain is not meaningless; it is meant to bring the initiate into a new state of being.

The ultimate initiation, both in myth and in practice, is dying and rising. In Christianity, we put people under the water in baptism, call it the "watery tomb," and bring them up as new creatures, children of God. Indigenous tribes have countless rites of passage in which they symbolically portray dying and rising. And the most ancient myths are full of these stories.

Finally, despite my difficulties with the Christian faith as a resource for this journey, I have discovered the priceless pearl in the middle of everything else: the death and resurrection of Jesus. My old self died, and I arose a new being. This is not the final initiation, of course, but there is no doubt I will have my turn at that one. Perhaps it will be a little easier because I have been initiated once already. We shall see.

FIVE

Do I Hold On
or Let Go?

Carol

Early on, my greatest fear was not that I might die of cancer, but that I had been responsible for it. When I finally rode out the waves of guilt and shame, I found myself in unexpectedly calm waters. Through the mastectomy and recovery from surgery and on into the early rounds of chemotherapy, often I felt God holding me. It was as if all my debts had been forgiven and I was at peace. But still, I did not want to die.

Somewhere between rounds three and four of chemotherapy, I went to see a healer. She was a wise, older woman—a midwife of the spirit— who put me into a state of deep relaxation. I had consulted with Em on and off since coming to Nashville. I had always trusted her with the most intimate secrets of my psyche when it came to relationships and career issues. Now the stakes were higher. In her low, soothing voice, she guided me to visualize myself eradicating the cancer cells. Nothing came to me. I simply could not visualize myself doing violence to the cells. She counted me down even deeper. Suddenly, I began to giggle. "What's happening?" she asked.

"I found a way to deal with them," I answered.

What had popped into my mind was the scene from *The Wizard of Oz* when Dorothy throws the water on the witch and she melts. But I didn't identify the cells with the witch. No, what came to my mind was that the cancer cells were like the witch's royal guards and winged monkeys. As the witch melted, I watched in pleasure as the cancer cells bowed down to me: "Hail, Carol. You killed the wicked witch. Hail, Carol!"

"You mean to say," Em finally responded, "that instead of killing your cancer cells, you are liberating them?"

"Looks like it!" I said, rather proud of myself.

"But Carol, you don't need to save your cancer cells, any more than you need to save the world."

"If I don't, who will?"

"Let God caretake your cancer cells so that you can focus your energy on healing yourself rather than on redeeming them."

We sat in silence. It made sense. But oddly enough, when I emerged from that session, the peace that had infused my life was no more. The intimacy with God was gone. Suddenly, I felt alone and scared. I came home to an empty house. The kids were at various after-school activities. There was a message on the answering machine that an emergency had come up at the office and Dan would not be home for dinner.

I seethed. Dan, who had been at my beck and call for months; who had dutifully volunteered for the task of giving me a daily shot needed to counteract the side effects of chemotherapy; who had stuck with me through it all—boy, was he going to get it when he came home. As promised, I sprang like a snake. "You are looking for an excuse not to come home," I hissed. "You're tired of taking care of me! Admit it!"

"Don't you dare talk that way to me," he replied, louder than a hiss.

"I'll talk to you however I damn well please!" I was screaming now.

"Then you can go to hell!" He shouted back.

Somewhere in the house a door slammed. As if we had been awakened by an alarm clock, we suddenly looked into each other's eyes and started laughing.

Why were we laughing?

Because you don't say "Go to hell" to a dying woman. He said it—so I must not be dying. With a few well-chosen swear words, I had turned the corner toward recovery.

The next time I saw Em, I told her what had happened. Even though on some deep level, I knew that my anger meant that I was getting better—I did not understand why I no longer felt as close to God as I had for many months. My anger was like a heat-seeking missile. After Dan, I had become angry with some of my dearest friends who invited themselves to the house for a healing service, and then expected me to lead it. Then, when my regular nurse was on vacation, her student replacement poked too hard and in the wrong place. Finally, my anger settled—and quietly remains—focused on the military-industrial complex, fueled by greed, machismo, and selfishness, that has polluted the environment and raised to unprecedented levels the risk for developing cancers. At least my anger is not often turned against myself.

Em explained to me that what I'd gotten those first peaceful few months was a kind of sneak-peek, sort of a spiritual "trying it on for size." The experience of serenity was real enough, I replied, in that if I had died, I would have died in peace. The thing is, I didn't die. It had become increasingly apparent to me that for the foreseeable future, I was going to live. In fact, I realized that I was going to live—as do we all—my entire life, however long that was. Now I was on the verge of discovering one of the world's greatest-kept secrets: It's easier to die than it is not to. You see, I had learned that I could, if necessary, die peacefully. But what was it going to take for me to pick up again the mainstream of my life?

I understand why so many people answer this question by going to war. Living through cancer is arduous. So is life. The temptation—healthy or ill—is to try to be strong all the time. But true power is about knowing when to push—and when to let go. Sometimes it is appropriate to struggle against the odds. Other times, it's about relaxing and allowing yourself to just be a sick person who has to rely on other people and other sources of strength.

Since the time of Dan's and my momentous argument, I began to have an expanded understanding about what it means to fulfill the human potential. It is not just about picking one note out of the spectrum of possibilities: peace or joy, power or faith. The juiciness of life comes from the complexity. The wrestling with paradox; bittersweet choices; even the broken hearts. Life is not a neat and tidy affair. If you want any of it, you need to take it all. And I wanted everything. With Dan's and my heated exchange of words, I was asking God to give me all my troubles back: cranky clients, traffic jams, spats with friends!

During this time of transition, I stumbled across a unique interpretation of the story of the sacrifice of Isaac in one of my textbooks. Do you remember the story from the Hebrew Scriptures? God tells Abraham he wants him to sacrifice his son Isaac. Abraham follows instructions, bringing Isaac to the mountain designated by God for the ritual slaughter. As Abraham and his young son walk up the mountain, Isaac keeps asking, "Where is the lamb for the sacrifice?" Abraham answers, "God will provide the lamb." When they get to the top of the mountain, Abraham prepares the altar for the sacrifice. Still no lamb. At last, Abraham binds Isaac to the altar and is about to kill him when an angel intervenes to stop him. Then Abraham discovers the sacrificial ram, horns tangled in the brambles nearby. Isaac was freed and the animal sacrificed in his place.

In the beginning, when I was first diagnosed with cancer, I felt that I understood this story as Abraham's test of faith. Abraham trusted God so much, he would even give up the life of his beloved son, if asked. Now I, too, was being tested. I was being asked to be willing to give up my own life, if asked. But what kind of a God would administer such a test?

Then I read the alternate interpretation of the story, the one I now choose to follow. There was a test, all right. But it was a test that Abraham flunked. God had wanted Abraham to say, "NO!" *No, I will not sacrifice my child. Life is too precious. I choose not to obey!* God had to send an angel to do what Abraham had not—stop the sacrifice and set Isaac free.

This second interpretation teaches us that God wants us to value life and to argue with our fate, especially when it is unjust. That was, in truth, what I had been doing from the beginning. It was I who, after all, walked myself in for a mammogram, rushed and rude as I was that day. Despite false starts and bad luck, I chose a doctor and treatments that would give me the best chance of recovery. I listened to my gut and turned to certain books for advice and inspiration and was quick to put others down. I let myself rest. I invited certain people into my inner circle and protected myself from others. I willingly suffered the pain of surgery and the discomfort of treatment, determined to do everything I could to give myself the best chance of living. Through it all, I kept opening myself to receive love and prayers and God's grace.

Every four months, I go to the doctor's office and get tested. They take my blood, they feel the glands in my neck. I am learning to receive test results as information—a life mandate, not a death sentence. *What do I need to do next to live as much life as I can fully, wholly, and deeply?* I now understand that my path is not to surrender passively to fate. But neither is it to fight against it. I have been blessed with a third choice: I can hope. No matter what, I can always hope. But to allow one's self to hope is to take a risk. And in taking this risk, I am living my life dangerously, indeed.

Susan

In the days and weeks after my diagnosis, I felt as if I were in a permanent state of free-fall. I had appointments with the surgeon, the oncologist, the radiologist, the anesthesiologist, and my primary care physician. I flailed around without moorings, and then BLAM! I landed in some strange spot, as if I had been spit out of a fun house chute. People seek these thrill rides to jolt themselves out of their normal perspectives. I had not chosen this adventure. I wanted it to go away.

Instead, my calendar filled with doctors' appointments, my conversations with worry, and my nights with fear. Day after day, I had to find another clinic, and give the same information for my chart that I had given a hundred times before. I am allergic to sulfa drugs. I take synthroid. My mother had breast cancer and is still alive. My grandmother died from breast cancer at age thirty-five. No, I do not smoke. Yes, I drink wine.

At first, it was not a question of letting go. That had already happened. I was trying to hold on. To what? To myself as a person, not myself as a disease. I wanted to have the best possible care from the medical system, but I did not want to be ground up and spit out as another statistic, one more patient on an assembly line.

This is a real tension for patients. Later, I took a close look at the information form used for patients at the breast center. There were large spaces for medical history and test results. The place to write in my social history was only one single-spaced line. Not even room for a paragraph to tell my entire story. No wonder I felt as if I were being squeezed into a convenient format and suspended from my life.

In order to be treated, I had to learn when to let go. I had to follow the rules, be on time for my appointments, and undress when asked. I had to let go of thinking of myself as a person in good health, for now I had cancer. I had to accept that I would lose a breast, although I could get a reconstructed version that looked good but had no feeling. There were so many little things. So much to let go.

With so much gone so swiftly, what was left to hold on to? My entire web of relationships was disrupted. Even with those I love and who love me, every relationship had to be reconsidered, realigned, and in some cases renegotiated. Would my husband run away from the difficulties ahead? Would he love me with a disfigured body? Would my children be terrified into silence, or turn to me for comfort? Would my friends pity me? Would I be forced out of my job?

As it turned out, I did not have to hold on. Instead, I was held. I was held in the arms of a loving family, caring friends, and thoughtful coworkers. I was touched, surprised, humbled, and moved to tears by an outpouring of kind gestures, practical help, and thoughtful advice. Had I not had cancer, I do not know if I ever would have glimpsed what has become the most cherished aspect of my life.

My treatment was successful, and my schedule returned to normal. Likewise, the cards, the flowers, the phone calls, and the dinners stopped. For family and friends, other worries became more pressing than my health. Not for me. This was the second time when the full impact of my illness hit. The first was my diagnosis. The second was after the commotion of treatment had ended. No doctor's appointments. No friends. Just me, back to my life, but the continuity had been severed. I felt as if I had lost my foundation.

I read a description of this phase as "crash and burn." Meditation helped me through this crisis. In addition to my own practice, I had the good fortune to find a "stress reduction" group based on the work of Jon Kabat-Zinn. The principles of this technique are gentle yoga stretches, silent meditation, and accepting what is.

I am pleased to say that this group is part of a conventional medical center, and I hope this is a trend. All patients should be offered these choices, therapies for the spirit and the body.

The beginning step of mediation is learning to be still. The next steps are watching the breath. Follow the breath on the inhalation. Follow the breath on the exhalation. In. Out. There is a feeling of contraction on the inhalation, and expansion during exhalation. After a time, when one learns to quiet the body and the mind, it seems as if there is only breath, as if the breath is breathing me instead of the other way around.

The secrets of life are told on the breath. On the exhalation the world is created. On the inhalation, everything is reabsorbed. There is all. There is nothing. There is life. There is death. Everything is held. Everything is let go. It is all the same, part of the mystery that is learned in the silence.

In dealing with cancer, I held on and I let go. Holding on and letting go complete the cycle of breath. Breath is not only my life, but life itself, the life I borrow for these sacred, precious years and return all too soon. *Breath* comes from the same root word as *spirit*. The essential practice of the spiritual path is not learned on a high mountain, in a cave, in a church, synagogue, or mosque. It is the practice of breath, our first act and our last, shared by all who live.

Linda

I have never viewed cancer as a battle.

It seemed to me that if I did not embrace it as a part of who I was, albeit a part that I wanted to change, then I could not recover. If I hated it, if I saw it as an enemy, then I would embark on an internal battle where there could be no victory.

In twelve-step philosophy, it is said that "there are no mistakes in God's world. . . . Acceptance is the answer to all my problems today."

The question for me was not do I fight or do I surrender, but do I live or do I die (in metaphorical terms, although it had a way of creeping in in a literal sense, sometimes).

The belief I had in acceptance had saved me many times, so I took it on faith that I could call it up once more. All it required of me was trust and showing up. Yes, the latter demanded a physical energy that chemotherapy had sucked out of me, but at least I didn't have to wake up every day, plot my strategy, and fight a battle with cancer.

What I did have to do was to let go, which is just a shade different from acceptance but a whole lot harder. In a war, when one side surrenders, they run a white flag up the pole and then the opposing generals get together and, I imagine, there is solemn backslapping along with insincere declarations: "Good fight, buddy. You're a worthy enemy."

It seems to me that letting go in your heart means something entirely different—it is part of a process, something that happens, not something that you set out and do.

If letting go were something you could choose to do, it's not likely you ever would. After all, our instinct is to fight—or to flee. When there is a diagnosis of illness that will change your life, that may even end your life, it is that instinct that we become aware of first. With either choice, we are taking action. It gives us a perception of control a moment after the words have shattered life as we know it, have broken what was whole and true into more fragments than we could have imagined.

Instinct says find every piece and get the strongest glue you can and put it all back together, no matter how hard you must struggle. I can make it just like it was, you think, just like it was. But you can't, of course, and so it is by going against everything that is natural that you find yourself hoisting that white flag in a place called Faith, a place where healing begins.

Karen

Many long years ago, I thought "surrender" to God was an act of will. I have discovered since cancer that it is really more a matter of giving up.

Surrender has a long and honorable tradition in Christian history. Many of the spiritual masters write about surrender. The ideal, of course, is Jesus in the Garden of Gethsemane: "Yet not what I want, but what you want." In the ideal, we are to be completely surrendered to God's will.

I live and work in the mainline church, and I have discovered that this view of surrender has had a terrible effect on people's prayer lives. I seem to end up leading a prayer group in whatever congregation I am in, and eventually we always come to this issue. People think that to pray "Thy will be done" means having none of their own. This simply is not the way things are.

The most telling example of that, again, is Jesus. In Gethsemane he did, in fact, surrender to God's will. But he also made it very plain what he wanted: "All things are possible for you. Take this cup away from me!" There was no doubt in his mind what outcome he desired. Jesus also taught his disciples the Lord's Prayer, which is really a list of requests.

I had to remind myself of all this constantly during my treatment. Especially after I went through the "Why me? Why not me?" questions, it seemed somehow wrong to ask for healing.

I think part of my fear about asking to live was fear of being disappointed. I was afraid God might not say "Yes" to my prayers—and then where would I be? Ironically, that is just what happened. I started begging to live the day I was diagnosed, but it took almost two years before it looked like I just might hang around a while. For a long time, it seemed as though I was on a fast track to death. Every treatment the doctors tried failed. And just as I had feared, I *was* disappointed with God. More than that—God felt like an enemy.

Cancer gave me bizarre literary tastes. I read Gerard Manley Hopkins every day:

Wert thou my enemy, O thou my friend,

How wouldst thou worse, I wonder, than thou dost
Defeat, thwart me? . . .

All the old-fashioned language aside, I like the sentiment: "God, if you were my enemy, I don't think you could hurt me worse than you do as my friend." I also liked Teresa of Avila's complaint to God: "No wonder you don't have many friends. Look at the way you treat the ones you *do* have." I would cry up to the sky, "How could things be worse if you were *trying* to make them bad?"

I ran into conservative Christians who told me that, in a sense, I was right about this. God was punishing me for my sins, whatever they were—and they were always very careful not to ask. Now, I will agree with them that I am a sinner. But the suffering I endured during treatment simply was not justified by my sins.

Besides, the Bible itself says this approach is misguided. The whole Book of Job insists that suffering is not necessarily connected to sin. Sometimes the innocent suffer. Very often, the sinful prosper. And then, of course, we have the example of Jesus. Completely without sin—that's what traditional Christianity teaches us—and yet he suffered.

All that said, it became an act of will to believe that God was on my side and not an enemy. I would say very calmly to myself and others that I believed God loved me and was working for the best in my life. I could not, though, *feel* that at all.

As I said, back in my romantic mystic-wannabe period, I thought surrender to God was an act of will. If I could just get to the right point of spiritual maturity, then I could turn my whole life over to God. But I discovered this is not how it works. Surrender has the meaning it does in war: I give up, God.

That is what it took, finally. I gave up and put my life in God's hands. If that meant death, then so it would be. The same if it meant life. Of course, this had always been the reality of my situation; by giving up, I simply stopped pretending I had any control over things.

I gave up because I was tired. I had done absolutely everything I knew how to do to get better. I had put myself under the care of one of the best oncologists in the country. I prayed regularly for healing. I had been anointed with oil, had hands laid on me, and had others pray for my healing. I tried to keep a positive attitude. I went to my support group as often as I could. But nothing I did seemed to make any difference. It seemed that with each doctor's appointment, the news got worse. So I gave up. I put my hands in the air and said, "All right, I give up. You are in charge of my future." I let go.

This is not at all to say that I did not have very strong feelings about what I *wanted.* I wanted to live. There was no doubt about that. Despite the fact that I felt rotten because of treatment, I wanted to live. Despite the fact that the end of my Ph.D. program was in sight and I could not get a job, I wanted to live. Even though I did not have a man in my life, I wanted to live. Even though my friends bailed out on me, I wanted to live. And I made sure God knew that. But I stopped trying to will my recovery into being. I stopped, in effect, trying to be God.

This is a posture that has served me well even since I have been in "remission." It is in my nature to be a control freak. That is a double problem because I am a competent person. There are many, many things in my life that I *can* control, whether by hard work, persuasion, or some other means. I still lapse into those old, bad habits on occasion. I know I am doing that, because along with the illusion of control comes incredible anxiety. And I strive to control the silliest things in my life. Cancer is a constant reminder not to travel down that path. A checkup, a treatment, a funeral insurance bill, or simply a pause to remember my situation rescues me from that drive for control.

Another misconception I had about surrender was that it is something we do once. That has not been my experience. Perhaps that just means I am not very spiritually mature. But for those of us who are spiritual babes, the fact seems to be that we must surrender again and again.

I know I will have more surrendering to do in the future. I have accepted my death, though I want to put it off as long as possible. But when I think about dying, I have very strong desires: I want to die at home, with people I love around me. I do not want to have pain. And yet my realistic side tells me I may not get what I want even when I am dying.

A psychiatrist I saw during my treatment assured me that cancer patients do not feel too much pain in the process of dying. He *insisted* that was so. "The brain knows what's going on," he said, "and it protects the person from horrible pain." But he is wrong. I did not know that at the time, although I suspected he did not know what he was talking about. Today, I have been at the bedsides of too many cancer patients in the end stages to believe him. Some of them do not have pain because of the type of cancer they have. Some of them have pain that is controlled by medication. But some of them have pain that persists despite the best efforts of medical science. The doctors kept one woman I know under general anesthesia for days at a time because that was the only way to keep the pain away.

I want to die at home, but the fact is I am a single woman whose family is scattered. Hospice is a wonderful organization, but for it to work, there must be a caregiver in the home twenty-four hours a day. I do not have anyone in my life who could do that. My sisters have their own families and could not leave their children for the months it would take me to die. It may be that I can go stay with my parents while I am dying. That takes me out of my own home, but it is better than the hospital. I have to realize, though, that at this writing my parents are in their mid-sixties and when the time comes, they simply may not have the physical stamina to keep me at their home. So I will probably end up in the hospital.

I do not want to die alone. A dear friend of mine from support group did, though. Another group member went by the hospital to see her and found her dead. The medical staff knew nothing about it. I have had the experience of friends fleeing from the terror of my illness; it is all too easy to imagine even more of them running away from the horror of death. Even if a cadre of family and friends kept a deathbed watch, there is always the possibility that I could die when someone goes to dinner or to the bathroom. It is entirely possible that at the moment I die, I will be alone.

I will fight to keep pain at bay, to stay at home, to have companions. The only one who can finally give me those gifts, though, is God. And while I am still working on it, at some level I have surrendered even these last wishes. If I do not get them, God will have to listen to my bitching and moaning through my last hour, but although I know very clearly what I want, I can, at base say, "Not what I want, but what you want."

SIX

Do I Trust the Medical Establishment or Do I Put My Faith in Alternative and Spiritual Healing?

Carol

My illness was like a rip in the fabric of our community. Many people came to do what they could to help mend it. Some carried casseroles. Others brought stories. One of the first stories I heard was from a business associate named Ellen. I had not known Ellen well before my diagnosis became public. An administrative assistant to one of our clients, she was one of the background people who wove in and out of my work life with pleasant enough greetings and polite responses. Our relationship was entirely by phone. I had never met her in person.

Nevertheless, when she heard about my illness, she asked to visit. She arrived at my home at a pivotal moment. Having already had the mastectomy, I was now preparing myself to enter the scary world of chemotherapy. I was sure I was doing the right thing, but I was also afraid and vulnerable.

Ellen arrived at the door, with long brown hair and earnest concern. She was rail thin and her complexion was disconcertedly pale. She had been one of the flower children from San Francisco who twenty years ago had followed her guru across the country to live on a hippie farming commune just outside of Nashville. Like many of the early settlers, she had over the years drifted away from the rigors of communal life to the luxury of a private bathroom in town with running water. Now she worked as a secretary at a mainstream company. But on the side, she peddled herbs.

We chatted casually, just long enough for her to ascertain that I had decided to undergo chemotherapy. Then she told me The Story.

The Story was about two friends from the commune, each of whom had been diagnosed with breast cancer. One of them had listened to her doctors and allowed them to cut into her body and poison her with chemicals. I will spare you the details of her complicated side effects, although I was not so lucky. Suffice it to say, the first one died. The other one had supposedly been diagnosed with an even more advanced stage of cancer. Rather than trust the medical establishment, she walked out of the doctor's office and put herself on an austere macrobiotic diet, meditated twice daily, bought a deionization machine, got herself rebirthed and acupunctured. And then there were herbs and huge amounts of filtered water and something about some pregnant animal's urine. She had figured out what the lesson of her cancer was, paid off her karmic debts, and gotten her energy flow reversed. The tumor cleared up, and though she'd never gone back to be examined, she knew she was now cancer free.

"Carol, walk out! Walk out now, while you still can! Don't let them poison you! There's a healthier way for you to go. I know—because I am the friend who lived."

I looked into Ellen's earnest deep-set eyes, her too-thin body—my fear fully ignited. By choosing chemotherapy, was I doing the right thing? As the daughter and daughter-in-law of two physicians and the sister of another, I was predisposed to putting my faith in traditional medicine. Before this, it never seriously occurred to me to turn my back on my physicians' recommendations for treatment, including chemotherapy. I trusted that the individuals in the medical establishment I had chosen to partner with were competent and caring. I wanted to take advantage of the cutting edge of what Western scientific research had learned about the human body.

But at the same time, I had for years been careful about what I put into my body. I avoided additives of all kinds. I ate whole grains and paid extra for organic vegetables. Now I was going to put poison into my veins? I shivered at the thought. Maybe Ellen was right. If I followed her recommended alternative course of treatment, I could be as healthy as she. But there was one problem. She did not look healthy. The tumor may have gone away, but there was something missing.

I took her pamphlets about herbs and supplements, psychic and emotional healings, and thanked her for coming. Instinctively, I knew that I was not going to take her advice and walk away from my doctor's care to be just like her. But it was several weeks, thinking about the incident on and off, before I knew what had been missing. Humility. That's what was missing from her earnest, deep-set eyes. She was so sure she had all the answers, not only for herself, but for me, too. In her desire to help me, she had dismissed my way as being the road to death. She was not interested in hearing what my intuition was telling me about my treatment. How I was being guided to trust my physicians. There was no space in her story where I could express my concern for her that she had not been recently tested; that she was not taking advantage of all her options for healing, including Western medicine.

When she left, the pile of brochures about herbs, supplements, and alternative treatments remained on the kitchen table. As much as I wanted to dismiss the extra layers of fear our exchange had generated in me, I could not bring myself to throw them out. There was a part of me that couldn't help thinking that there was something in all this. Sure, a lot of it was nonsense. But what if there was some herb, some alternative treatment, that smarter, wiser, luckier people knew about? I decided to talk to my doctor about it.

"There is no scientific evidence that any of these remedies provide the results your friend promised," he said. "But I would have no problem if you wanted to add some in. The ones you've told me about certainly won't do you any harm."

I nearly ran home to the stack of brochures, pen and checkbook in hand, to place my order. But which ones were smoke and mirrors,which ones contained truth? If I'd ordered everything she'd recommended, I could have opened my own pharmacy. And, too, while I could conceivably take a loan to pay for everything she told me to do, I would find myself rushing from one healer to another, pressed for time. There wouldn't have been time to rest and heal. Under the circumstances, too much seemed as risky as too little.

I went to see my spiritual advisor, Em.

She listened to my story then smiled.

"Ah! You're in the magic bullet stage," she offered.

"What's that?"

"That desperate moment when you think if only you could get it exactly right, you could be in complete control of your destiny."

"Shouldn't I do everything I can within my power to heal myself of cancer?" I asked.

"Yes, but 'everything' includes taking the time to listen to your own intuition. Get quiet enough, and you will know what to do."

"But I can't afford to waste any time with this."

She looked at me, nodding wisely. "I see. You think it's all up to you. You've lost faith in your body's willingness to heal itself—and you are forgetting God's ability to transcend whatever 'mistakes' you make. If you really trusted God, you would be free to take a less frantic, driven approach to your healing. You could try things out, experiment gently with various combinations of herbs and treatments. Keep the ones that feel right—move on from those that don't. I know that you would prefer to take matters into your own hands and do exactly what you need to heal perfectly. But what if you followed my advice, relaxed into your decision-making process, and settled for a 'B' rather than an 'A' in healing?"

I have been accused of being a perfectionist before. As we sat quietly together, I found myself thinking about Ellen. Her austere mission had given her a sense of mastery in her life—but at the expense of her own vitality. I was beginning to make the connection between humility and healing. Then Em shared something with me she'd never told me before.

"Eighteen years ago, I got a tumor on my spine. The doctor told me I needed surgery. But I refused his recommendation. Instead, for ten years, I followed every alternative therapy I could get my hands on. I used herbs, I meditated, I went to an acupuncturist, I underwent hypnotherapy. I got amazing insights from my healing process—the tumor gave me incredible gifts."

"And then it cleared up?" I offered.

"No. For ten years, I got every kind of mental, physical, and spiritual lesson you could possibly get from a tumor, and still it didn't go away. Finally, I said 'Oh, hell,' and got the damn thing out."

This was not the ending I'd expected. In truth, it was much greater, for it reminded me that even among the best of us, we are all still human. We can do all we can within our financial, emotional, and physical means to heal ourselves. We can make use of traditional and alternative therapies. But the most important thing we can do is to stand back in awe of the miracle of healing that is always possible, trusting that this can happen at any time and in any way, regardless of what we are or are not doing. When I consider my options, I ask myself this key question: "Will this support my innate capacity to heal, understanding that with God's help, I am already healing?"

Ultimately, I put my faith neither fully in traditional medicine nor in alternative therapies. Rather, I put my faith in God.

Linda

The first oncologist I saw was really a jerk.

There, I've said it—disrespectful words about a doctor—and I have no regrets.

After diagnosis of any life-threatening illness, you quickly can be caught up in what can be a medical nightmare. If I can tell you anything to help you face that challenge, it is this: "Slow down. This is about your life. Ask questions. Listen to the answers. If you don't like the responses you are getting from one doctor, say, "Thanks, but no thanks." You are about to embark on a road filled with unimaginable terrors; you don't want to make the trip with someone who won't listen to you."

So I didn't. After walking out on the jerk, I asked for recommendations from other people—other doctors and nurses, as well as from friends. What I ended up with was a team of highly skilled professionals who still had time to listen.

Every doctor that I saw—the general surgeon, the plastic surgeon, the medical oncologist, the radiation oncologist—always included heartfelt questions: "How are *you*? How are you doing emotionally?"

From the beginning, it was very important for me not to lose myself and become only a cancer patient, and the medical team I chose understood and respected that need. So did my friends, my therapy group and its leaders, my family, my neighbors, my coworkers.

And although I was not *just* a cancer patient, the fact remained that I was still a cancer patient. One of the things that means is that you have to make a lot of medical choices, and none of them is going to be really fun.

For a growing number of women who have breast cancer that requires surgery, there is a choice between a mastectomy or a lumpectomy.

That choice got eliminated right away for me, because I had what one doctor said was "a really nasty tumor"—a frank assessment of a cancerous mass with more tentacles than an octopus, reaching out from its hiding place beneath my breastbone and trying to hang on to the pectoral muscle, the chest wall, anything it could grab. It cost me a breast and a big chunk of lymph nodes, but the former was replaced with a brand new breast—sort of—reconstructed from abdominal tissue.

Five days after surgery I went home sprouting clear plastic tubing and reservoir-type bulbs, two in my chest and two in my abdomen, to drain incisions. The unfamiliar quickly became routine, as I emptied the bulbs of the mixture of blood and other fluids, measured and recorded the amounts, and changed portions of the dressings.

Beneath my growing familiarity with the wounds, however, I had increasing apprehension about what was ahead.

During the surgery, a portion of tissue that contains lymph nodes was removed from the hollow of my left armpit. When a cancer has metastasized, or spread, it is often present in the lymph nodes near the original tumor site.

The severity is measured, in part, by "positive nodes," that is, the presence of cancer outside the tumor site. When I read the pathology report suggesting a small amount of "metastatic mammary carcinoma," I began talking to the runaway cancer cells: "What did you run for? Why didn't you stay with all those other bad cells?" And then I began to beg: "Stop, please. Don't spread."

I tried to stay centered and calm, but the inner voices were not always cooperative. Repeatedly they cried out in agony, and sometimes yours will, too. If our spirits are not passionately aware, whether in angst or joy, we are missing a great deal in life.

Even though it was painful, I also considered my mortality. I understood that the diagnosis meant a heightened possibility that I would not reach the biblical "threescore years and ten," or whatever contemporary life span predictions are.

I also realized that I loved my life—my family, my friends, my job. Even considering that my life might be shortened, I didn't feel the need to make dramatic changes, to do anything differently.

But then there was chemotherapy, which quickly began to make dramatic changes. I was about to learn, like so many before me, that the trick is not to survive cancer, it's to survive treatment. Some people call the standard medical protocol for treating cancer "slash, poison, and burn," for surgery, chemotherapy, and radiation. I have to admit that at my lowest points, I absolutely agreed. Still, for me, I preferred to take my chances there instead of seeking out herbalists, acupuncturists, and others who offered alternative therapies.

But that is not to say that I believed medicine would provide a cure. On the contrary, I believed that by turning the care of my physical body over to physicians, nurses, and other medical personnel whom I trusted, it would allow me to focus on the mental, spiritual, and emotional aspects of recovery.

That is the way I found to go beyond the illness, to a place where I believe true healing is possible.

But first I had to open the door.

On the side where I stood, I gave lip service to spirituality. I used my head to talk about my heart.

In fact, in the conversation with the surgeon following my biopsy—while I was still groggy and in the recovery room—I told her, basically, that this was going to be a piece of cake.

I ticked off what I'd already mastered—difficult childhood, alcohol and drug abuse, divorce—and assured her that I was totally prepared to take cancer into my life and make lemonade.

I was wrong, and I am grateful for that.

In the past, I had no qualms about trying to leap tall buildings in a single bound—I took pride in super-strength. I tried hard. Very hard.

What I learned when my life was threatened by illness was that I had to give up trying, slow the activity and effort. I had to push open a door and walk into the dark night of the soul, with no map, no light, and no turning back.

Oh, yes, I kept showing up for myriad medical appointments, but I was armed with increasing calmness, not a thousand questions for which the only answers began with "One in four breast cancer patients. . . ."

In my heart I was moving on, moving away from self-will and toward what I hoped would be acceptance.

In the midst of treatment—you're sick, you're tired, you're bald—it is not easy to put your mind at rest. But because I chose to let the doctors practice medicine, I could detach from the assault of information coming at me from the media and from well-meaning friends. It was my decision not to tap into my extremely limited well of energy to look at the latest results of Tamoxifen studies, or the benefits of essiac tea or burdock root.

By accepting without question the help of the medical establishment, I was taking a chance—a chance that maybe my doctors didn't have the information that would be best for me, that perhaps they had an agenda that was contrary to what I believed. Still, there was a choice to make, and I made the one that I could by acknowledging that peace and harmony were attainable. In the natural order of things, I might die sooner rather than later, and there was nothing I could do that would, with certainty, prevent that.

Until I was faced with cancer, I had spent my life doing, rather than being. I thought if I learned more, I would achieve intellectual success; if I acquired more, I would have material wealth.

So while the doctors in whom I had put my trust were gathering information, I was giving it up. Instinctively, I was led by Eastern thought from the *I Ching*. I had to accept that in order to achieve wholeness, I would first have to be incomplete, and that before I would be reborn to a new life, I would have to experience, metaphorically, the death of the old one.

Spiritually, that's the state I hoped to attain; but physically, I kept getting poison injected into my veins. After all, even philosophers sometimes hedge their bets.

Have I kept the peace?

The answer would have to be, "Sometimes." Almost five years out from treatment, when a CT scan showed an ovarian mass, there were a few hours of panic, followed by an overwhelming sadness, then bargaining—"If I don't die now, I'll be better, work harder, lose weight, eat more cruciferous vegetables...."

But by the time another battery of tests revealed that somehow my ovary, withered from chemotherapy, had managed to resurrect enough life to form a cyst, I had come to terms with what might be, and was truly grateful for those five years.

I have no regrets about the path I chose, medically or spiritually. Yes, sometimes I look at the photographs that were made of my breasts before the mastectomy, before a dozen more surgeries to strip away muscle, rebuild a breast, and examine new growths that the doctors deemed "suspicious." But in those pictures, and in the mirror, I see the body I have today, bearing its scars like a road map to a place called Serenity, a resting place on the road to Peace.

Karen

It is responsible of me to arrange my funeral, given my prognosis. I am happy to say that I did that once, when I was living in Nashville, and have never needed it. So after I settled in Springfield, Tennessee, I went to a funeral home here. Since this is a small town, I called one of the owners of the funeral home, who invited me over that very afternoon. He met with me briefly and then turned me over to a woman on the staff whose sole job is "pre-need arrangements."

We went through what I wanted for the funeral, she calculated a price, and spent some time on the phone finding a company that would insure my funeral. All this took some time, and as it passed she learned about my situation. Finally our business was at an end, but as I stood to go, she called another woman in her tiny office and closed the door. "You can't say a word about this to anyone," she told me, "or I could lose my job." In the few seconds before she went on, I imagined all sorts of bizarre suggestions. What she and her friend had to say to me, though, was this: They both went to a doctor in Alabama who used herbs and some kind of light source to heal. They both knew women who had been diagnosed with incurable cancer and had been cured. The first woman pressed the doctor's name and telephone number into my hand, they both hugged me, and put the finishing touch on this astonishing encounter: They told me if I wanted to go and did not have the money, they would pay for it. I stammered my thanks and got out the door as fast as I could.

Had I been in a big city, I would have marched straight into the office of my friend, the funeral director, and told him all about this. But since I live in a small town, such actions could have lifelong ramifications not only for the women but for their whole circle of family and friends—some of whom are bound to be in my congregation. So I kept my peace.

Yet later, when I was telling friends about this bizarre offer, I found myself becoming more and more angry. As I said, it is responsible of me to arrange my funeral, and when I went I was in quite good health. But it still was not an easy thing to do. I was in a very vulnerable state, and these women ganged up on me and pressed me to avail myself of a particular alternative medicine.

This is not at all unusual. I have had countless people send me magazine articles and books and newspaper clippings about the latest miracle "cure" for cancer. I have received information on herbs, healing touch, aromatherapy, visualization, shark cartilage, apricot pits, and on and on and on. I am not the only person this happens to. A newly diagnosed friend got a telephone call from someone he barely knew. She told him not to make a move until he had talked to her. She insisted that radiation was only going to destroy his immune system, and she could cure him with the right diet.

People do this out of kindness and concern, I know. They care about me, and if there is some obscure treatment that the medical establishment has ignored, they want to be sure I have heard of it and can benefit from it. What they do not seem to realize is that, first of all, they are implicitly questioning the wisdom of the treatment route I have taken. We all must decide what kind of treatment—or lack of treatment—is right for us. Assuming that someone with cancer is an adult (and I am certainly way past that), the choice of treatment is his or her own decision. It is insulting, in a way, to suggest I do not know what I am doing given the choices I have made.

The fact is, of course, that there is a reason "slash, burn, and poison" is the conventional treatment for cancer: scientific studies have shown these are the most effective. That is why I have chosen them. I want the best odds I can get. And unfortunately, scientific studies have not shown that shark cartilage is helpful at all.

But what if *the* cure is out there and I just ignore it? What if the scientific community simply has not gotten around to testing how effective a particular herb is? Here is the problem, though: How do I choose among all the alternative treatments out there? How do I know that one or the other will work the magic? Suddenly I have become responsible for my cancer again. If I do not get well, it is because I have chosen the wrong kind of treatment. And except for conventional therapies, I have nothing to guide me. Every ad I have ever seen for these products has someone who *swears* he or she had incurable cancer and then got better after taking this treatment. I am not even skeptical about their claims. It is just that there is no guarantee that this particular alternative treatment is what brought about the cure. The only way to know that is through science, and then we are back to the original problem.

There was a time when I was vulnerable to the claims of alternative treatments. I think as human beings, we all have some paranoia, and Americans are particularly prone to believe in conspiracy theories. So it was not really a surprise when I first heard some cancer patients wondering whether the cure for cancer had already been discovered, and the medical establishment kept it hush-hush because otherwise they would all be out of jobs. This idea had already occurred to me. I think it is fair to speak of cancer treatment as an "industry," one that I imagine runs into billions of dollars each year. And what *would* all those oncologists do if cancer was easily curable? What would the cancer drug companies do? What would happen to all those cancer centers, all those expensive radiation machines, all that stockpiled Yew tree-derived Taxol at $3,000 a dose?

I got out of this conspiracy frame of mind by using my head. First of all, most conspiracies turn out to be a lot of bunk. Then there was my own oncologist, David Johnson. He has had cancer himself, and I cannot believe he would hide such knowledge. I know that since I have had cancer, I would do anything I could to prevent it, even in the people who have hurt me the most. The final reason, though, was the strongest: Doctors and researchers are not known for their small egos, and if someone had discovered a cure for cancer, she would have published it as soon as possible to get her Nobel Prize and her picture on the cover of the newsweeklies.

Most ministers in mainline Christian denominations believe that God heals through modern medicine. I heartily endorse that sentiment myself. It makes sense to me to say that God has given human beings the intelligence, the curiosity, and the altruism to discover cures for physical illnesses. Most of the time, at least, God seems to work through these conventional means. I have met more than one physician who says his or her ability to heal is, at base, grounded in the power of God. It is reasonable, then, from my theological perspective, to avail myself of the treatments available from the medical establishment. God is the great physician, but she has appointed doctors and nurses here on Earth to do most of her healing work.

My colleagues in the mainline churches would be comfortable with all I have just said. But they would, I am afraid, squirm when they heard my belief that God also heals directly through prayer.

There are many good reasons to believe in miraculous healing. One of Jesus' main activities, aside from delivering stirring speeches, was miraculously healing people. The apostles apparently carried on this work, according to Acts. The history of the church is full of stories of unexplainable cures. Pentecostal churches today claim myriad healings. But the final reason I believe in direct divine healing is that I have seen it myself. Most ministers, if questioned, will admit they have witnessed such things, but they rarely speak about it without prodding. Such things are downright embarrassing in the modern world.

I have seen two instances of God's healing. One was a little girl who had an inoperable brain tumor. While they could not save her life, the surgeons believed they could prolong it by removing much of the tumor mass. I sat with the family during the surgery, and after several hours the doctor came out with a copy of the CT scan taken several days before the operation. He said, "It's not there. The tumor's gone. I can't understand it. It must be . . . God." He said this with quite a bit of distaste.

The other instance was much closer to home. My beloved Aunt Evonne was diagnosed with pancreatic cancer in its earliest stage. There is no cure for cancer of the pancreas, and it is a particularly fast-growing type of cancer. The doctors told her she might have six months, but it would be wiser to count on six weeks. So she went ahead and let them take her pancreas out, refused all other treatment, and went home to die. She called Hospice and invited them in to help her and her family deal with her death. She knew she would not be around the next Christmas, so she went shopping and bought special gifts for everyone in our extended family. Six weeks came and went, as did six months. She just did not die. In fact, she did not die for another ten years. This was a mystery to her physicians, and they wanted to cut her open to see what was going on inside of her. She declined. The people in her church rejoiced, because they had been holding prayer vigils since she was diagnosed.

Neither of these cases is explainable by modern science. In neither of these cases did the patient take any alternative treatments. What they both had was prayer, and lots of it. And so when it came time for me to decide what treatment route I wanted to take, I decided on two paths: conventional medicine and prayer. I was even a bit stubborn about this. After I learned that my cancer had metastasized and was incurable, I refused to even consider something besides these two options. I told people, "If I survive, I want people to know it's because of God."

In the worst time during my illness, when several treatments had failed and the doctor said I might have only six months to live, I traveled to Lexington, Kentucky, to visit a dear friend of mine, a former seminary professor. While I had been in school, we had both been regulars at the 7 A.M. Eucharist celebrated by a tiny group of Episcopal nuns in a house next door to the seminary. I joined them for communion one morning during my visit, and after that short service was over, I knelt down. My friend anointed me with oil, laid hands on my head, and prayed for my physical healing. It was a very Episcopal service—quiet and dignified. There was no screaming, no being "slain in the spirit," no extravagant claims. Everyone in that room believed that God could cure me through prayer, and I must report that it was from that day I started getting better.

There is a huge claim implicit in that statement. I am not saying God *cured* me—she did not. I still have terminal cancer. But I am in a very unusual state of quasi-remission, a state my oncologist cannot understand. What I am saying is that God brought me back to health, and has kept me here for much longer than anyone has expected. My oncologist, who by his own account is not a religious man, calls me his "miracle patient."

I cannot explain this. I make no claims for special status with God. In fact, I am mystified; I do not understand why I have had this healthy time when other people have died quickly. I do not understand it at all. I only know it has happened.

And so I am very old-fashioned when it comes to my choices of treatment. I chose—and will choose in the future—medicine and prayer. I have no doubts there are other good choices out there, but these are mine.

Susan

Trusting the medical establishment was a central issue in my cancer treatment. I wanted to go to the finest scientific medical facility and learned that our university cancer center had the prestigious seal of approval from the National Cancer Institute. It is the only one in our region.

Like a tracker, I was looking for a sign. Prestige is not enough. Could I trust these people? A surgeon would be in charge of my care. I had never been to a surgeon. I could not shake my initial fantasies of men who cut women open with knives.

One problem in modern medicine comes from its advancements. Diagnostic tests can detect cancer long before the body feels anything. If something is wrong, I should be able to feel it. As I sit here writing, my chin itches wildly with an annual summer case of poison ivy. Red welts make their way from bump to blister. I wake up in the night wanting to scratch. I have all the signs of "something is wrong with me."

When I was diagnosed with cancer, I was feeling fine. The nurses and doctors located a thickening in my left breast, but only after they saw the telltale star shaped shadow on the mammogram. They guided my hand to the spot. From reading all those breast self-exam cards that I was supposed to hang in my shower, I thought I would feel a chickpea. It felt more like a pulled tendon.

So this was breast cancer? In the days before mammography, with my slow-growing cancer, I might have gone on living, never knowing that anything was wrong. Cancer entered my life as a disembodied concept. I was shocked and disoriented. My world had changed, not because of an accident or heart attack, but because of a conversation. Was this information true? Suppose they were wrong?

I did not know anyone at my local Breast Center. I never had to. Every year I went for my mammogram, hoping that the mammo-tech would be a good one. Some make the experience of breast-squashed-in-a-square-plastic-vice more pleasant than others. But trust? No need. Mammograms are not life-threatening. They are impersonal. Sidling up to the machine in a contorted position. Wondering what it is like to look at women's breasts all day. Waiting until the unseen radiologist says the films are readable. If they are, I am dismissed. Good-bye folks, until next year.

A suspicious mammogram, that star-shaped shadow in the midst of gray squiggles, changes the course of events. Instead of hearing nothing until next year, the phone call comes. More clinic visits. More tests. Fine needle aspirations. Biopsies. A close look at the cells inside the tumor. And those words, *You have cancer.*

Carol had an unfortunate first impression of my surgeon, compounded by summer vacations and lost records. After the mix-up, she switched to a different medical center. I stayed as his patient against her advice. I remained suspicious, even though he was clearly an expert. I tried to find out more about him, with methods most people use but may not admit. He was too new in town for grapevine gossip. He failed my East Coast Snob Test because he hadn't gone to Harvard. He was professional and reserved, veiling clues to his personality. What was I to do?

Meanwhile, at each appointment I looked around at the setting. What were these big machines, these white coats, these antiseptic smells, these uncomfortable tables and bright lights? They looked frighteningly close to instruments of torture. Inside the health care system, they are regarded as tools of healing. An outsider has no such context.

Healing should be comforting, warm, and smell good, like the embrace of a kind mother. I think this is one of the primary reasons why people seek alternative treatments. The settings for many of these treatments fit the archetype of a healing atmosphere: soft lighting and colors, good smells, individualized and attentive care from the moment a person enters the door.

Do alternative treatments work? In the Western scientific paradigm of randomized trials, we do not know. Little research has been done on their effectiveness. Thankfully, the approaches of traditional and alternative medicine are coming closer together. For example, UCSF Stanford Complementary Medical Clinic recently opened where they not only offer alternative treatments but will also study their effectiveness.

For a person with cancer or any life-threatening illness, this is wonderful news. Many people seek alternative treatments in secret, afraid that their physicians will not approve. Healing options will improve when traditional and alternative medicine respect one another and the person who is ill can choose the best from both.

With cancer there is so much uncertainty that trust became my only solid ground. The first person I had to trust was my surgeon. I had observed his thoughtful, serious manner, especially during medical procedures. He was gracious in answering my hundreds of questions, and in explaining his reasoning. I was waiting for reassurance that he was a decent human being.

The breakthrough came when I discovered we had a mutual friend. She told me he was an outstanding surgeon, and a loving husband and father. This was the kind of information I needed, not his credentials. This valuing of relationship over credentials is sometimes called women's way of knowing. Perhaps it comes more naturally to women, but all people use this test. However, not all people have access to this reassurance. This lack of trust discourages people from seeking medical care. For example, many women refuse to get screening mammograms, even though early detection of cancer may save their lives.

My trust opened some unforeseen doors. When Carol's breast cancer was discovered, her new doctor was unresponsive and cavalier. Observing the care I was receiving, she returned to my surgeon and medical center. Her cancer treatment was more extensive than mine. I hate to think what would have happened to her, had not my trust paved the way.

A second door opened, in part because of my initial sense of distrust. I showed my journals to my surgeon, uncensored writings about what it felt like to be his patient. He became curious, rather than defensive, and saw an opportunity to improve. For a year, we had a dialogue about how to bridge the great divide between doctors and patients. As I got to know him, I discovered the depth of his dedication and compassion, and was ashamed about my first impressions. When I apologized, he said not to worry. However it happened, I had found a way to trust, which he regards as essential in the doctor-patient relationship.

We are publishing our story, and hope it will offer insights for patients and doctors who wish to become partners instead of adversaries. Part of trust is learning to speak each other's language, and trying to see through each other's eyes.

I wish I could give some simple advice about trust. It is mutual. It requires effort, consideration, patience, and is not automatic. There are compassionate, trustworthy people everywhere. They may be in large, cold medical centers or in warm, incense-filled rooms. Trustworthiness is not a static state, but a quality that develops, and requires attention.

Learning to trust was a humbling lesson. It tested my spiritual ideals. Trust in God means trust in people. There are no rubrics to follow. It is a test of the heart.

Trust is the beginning of spiritual healing. It moves treatment to the realm of relationships, to compassion and love, the source of healing and care. The prophet Mohammed said, "Trust in God, but tie your camel." With trust, the science of medicine becomes a healing art.

Community

THE STAGE OF COMMUNITY MOST OFTEN BEGINS when acute treatment ends. This landmark is often missed because it would seem that the end of treatment is a time to rejoice. It's the time when the psychological and spiritual demons hit with great force. Treatment, however dreadful, is a kind of support system. When treatment ends, we are cut loose on all sides. We must recover from treatment, and put our lives back together. During this period, a supportive community makes all the difference.

Here are some of the questions we ask at this stage: From whom must I learn to receive? From whom must I learn to protect myself? In this stage we learn to trust our intuition. We must accept that some influences may be harmful, and we must weed these out. One of the most difficult things is to ask for what we need. Like treatment, there is no one way. Support comes in many forms. For example, traditional support groups work wonders for some women and are traumatic for others. Find what works for you.

Your friends and family can help by realizing that just

because treatment has ended, cancer is not over for you. They can stay with you for the ups and downs.

The more faithfully you listen to the voice within you,
the better you will hear what is sounding outside.
And only she who listens can speak.
—DAG HAMMARSKJOLD

A breast cancer diagnosis thrusts you into the center of frenzied activity. You are a rip in the fabric of the community. Some will rush in to fix the tear. Others will be repelled. Of those who come to help, some will be angels bearing gifts of love and light. Others will be misguided, inadvertently chipping away at your personal power and increasing your sense of guilt.

It is possible however, and necessary if you are to maintain emotional and spiritual centeredness, to learn not only how to receive, but also from whom to receive at such a vulnerable moment. When we share our experiences, it is our hope that we may empower others faced with similar situations to make better decisions about who they let in to help and how, and also to help friends, family, and acquaintances find the right words to truly be of service.

SEVEN

From Whom Must I Learn to Receive? From Whom Must I Learn to Protect Myself?

Carol

You will read between the lines of my story about the many people who gave freely to me of their love, their wisdom, and their caring. It was difficult at first for me to receive their gifts of time and friendship. For the first few weeks, I kept track of every flower bouquet, every casserole, every favor, feeling the growing pressure to pay it all back in kind as soon as I was able. As the goodness mounted, I felt less and less adequate to respond. How could I ever repay Jody's school guidance counselor, who personally brought Jody from school to visit me after my operation? My classmate who organized the student body to take turns providing meals for my family? Then Em came to visit. She heard me out, then quietly suggested that this was one of those times in life when you can and should just take it all in—no guilt, no obligation, no pressure. Relax and enjoy receiving the outpouring of love.

It was a tremendously liberating notion. I indulged myself on a test basis to see how it felt to receive unconditionally. Someone called to express her concern for me. I didn't call back for several days. A friend took Jody to the movies one dreary weekend. I didn't worry about what I could do in return. How did it feel? It felt just fine.

Of course, there can always be too much—even of a good thing like opening to receive love unconditionally. So many people came to see me in the hospital after my mastectomy, I could not get adequate rest. We gossiped and talked philosophy. Some rubbed my feet or offered helpful medical advice. The night before my eagerly awaited release from the hospital, the room full of visitors, I felt my temperature suddenly soar. If I were to get an infection, not only would it be dangerous to my health— but I would not be able to return home the next day, as planned. Seeing my distress, Dan cleared the room and sat quietly with me, holding my hand and dabbing my brow with a cool cloth. By the time the nurse came around to take my temperature, it had returned to normal. I had to learn to protect myself, even from the people who loved me.

Strangers, too. I was constantly challenged by well-meaning individuals who offered me the illusory promise of personal power in exchange for my humble faith. Just use this herb, that therapy—try to be smart and good enough—and you will be among the winners!

Even though I'd read the statistics reporting that individuals who attended cancer support groups outlive those who do not, I also had to protect myself from my fellow cancer patients. Not that they intended any harm. But it was my tendency to wear myself out (and then my doctors) pursuing any promising development in cancer treatment to emerge from somebody's mouth, even if the cure had only worked on a mouse and was years away from application to humans. At the same time, even a casual mention of any symptom I had not yet developed automatically put me on red alert. Sally felt soreness in this or that part of her body before her recurrence was diagnosed, and I would spend the next week palpating the corresponding portion of my anatomy ten times a day until the next, scarier symptom got mentioned in passing. After hearing about a certain symptom at a support group, one of my friends became so concerned about a red spot on her chest that she convinced her doctor to biopsy it. Turned out to be a bug bite. I came out of the meetings drained rather than bolstered, statistics notwithstanding.

Challenging as it was, the people in all of these categories were, if not well-meaning, at least neutral. But of course, there were some people who didn't like me all that much before I got breast cancer. And they didn't like me any better when I did. In fact, the people who were most adept at spreading the news of my difficulty were those who I least trusted to have my best welfare in mind.

Take Bonnie, for instance. When I'd first moved to Nashville, she befriended me. An active figure in the business community, she introduced me around and got me involved in some important organizations. Then we had a falling out. I'll spare you the details. Suffice it to say that I was right and she was wrong. We went our separate ways, as much as possible in a community as small as Nashville.

Then came the annual meeting for one of the key organizations with which, on her advice, I'd become involved. A little over halfway through my chemotherapy, I was feeling stronger and stronger. Free of any signs of cancer, a braver person would have called herself "cured." I simply reported to the gaggle of acquaintances who greeted me warmly at this meeting that "my prognosis is excellent." I took my seat in the back of the banquet hall, savoring the joy of small talk and chocolate tarts. So pleased was I to be back in the swing of things, I had completely forgotten that there was no hair under my attractive hat and that my eyebrows had been painted on.

The program began. The president made some remarks. Before long, it was time to award "Member of the Year." It wouldn't be me, as I had avoided any responsibilities in this particular organization. I settled back, content to simply be there and not stuck in some clinic somewhere. Then they called out Bonnie's name. She had won the award.

Seated on the far side of the banquet hall, I watched her shaking hands and smiling broadly as she made her way to the podium to accept. Bonnie stood at the dais, award in hand, scanning the hall. The applause died down. Then, after many, long moments, she said in hushed tones, "I'd like to dedicate this award to my dear friend Carol Orsborn, who is in a life and death struggle with breast cancer. If we might take a moment to offer up a silent prayer for Carol's recovery."

You might just as well have broadsided me with a truck. A few minutes earlier, I had been rolling the smooth pleasure of chocolate custard between my lips, now I was declared to be on death's doorstep. Bonnie went on to discuss my various contributions and virtues. The more she raved, the smaller I felt. This was it: I was attending my own funeral. But the eulogy was being given by someone I could not stand! Months later, I still bumped into people who thought that I'd died.

There's not much you can do to protect yourself from those individuals who didn't like you in the first place. But most people don't mean to be rude or intrusive. In fact, as I greet newcomers to the breast cancer world, I often find myself with two left feet, saying things I don't mean and meaning things I don't say. Dealing with mortality is awkward, at best. But there are some general guidelines. To help refresh myself before offering my support and friendship to a new recruit, I reread the following set of guidelines, written in the middle of my chemotherapy when people's helpful and hurtful responses were still fresh in my mind.

Things Not to Do
When Somebody You Care about Is
Diagnosed with a Serious Illness

• *Do not ask, "How are you?"*

How do you think they are? You already know they've got something serious. Why are you asking? What are you going to do with the information? When they hear these words from you, what they will really be hearing is this: "Are you going to die soon?" If you don't already know the details of their illness, you probably don't need to know.

If you are looking for a conversation starter, instead say, "It's great to see you!" Or, "I've been thinking about you a lot lately."

If you mean it, go on and ask a much better question: "Is there anything I can do?" Then offer something specific. Say, "Could you use help driving your daughter to her lessons?" or "May I bring you dinner tonight?"

- *Do not offer unsolicited medical advice.*

  You may be burning to share your theory about which hospital is the best, which drugs or therapy saved Aunt Bea's life. But before you blurt it out, ask your friend's permission. For instance, you can say—in a non-leading way—"Are you happy with your hospital?" If they are, then button it up. If not, you can ask, "Would you like me to do some research on other possibilities, or offer you some suggestions?"

- *Do not theorize on why your friend created his or her illness.*

  Unless there's scientific evidence—and something your friend can do about it now—keep your theories to yourself. While we're at it, don't call the cancer a "gift" or a "lesson." If they think of it that way for themselves, great! But if you say it about them, it comes off as patronizing at best. Think about it: Did they need this great gift or lesson more than you or anybody else? And please do not say, "God must love you very much."

- *Do not pay a visit and expect to be entertained.*

  Make it clear that you are going to be bringing along a treat for the patient (and/or his or her family) to enjoy. Come prepared with something upbeat or interesting to talk about. Do not succumb to the temptation to use the immobile patient as your sounding board or therapist. Remember that you are coming to give, not to get.

- *Don't:*

  Stay too long when your friend needs to rest.

  Expect return phone calls. Instead, leave messages that say, "I want you to know that I'm thinking about you. No need to call me back. But if you need anything, let me know and I'll be right over!"

Don't bring meals in pans that will need to be returned.

• *And my personal favorite:*

Under no circumstances may you eulogize somebody's illness publicly without first getting their permission.

Linda

When people ask me what the hardest part of facing cancer was, I reply with certainty, "Telling my parents."

I cannot tell you why, only that it would break their hearts; although we'd had our difficulties, I had somehow managed to get this far without doing that, either unavoidably or by my own choices.

On Sunday morning, two days after the biopsy had revealed an infiltrating breast cancer, I drove to their home a hundred miles from mine. My mother was cooking lunch and my father had gone to church. I wanted to tell them both at the same time; now I would have to wait.

I was suddenly angry: "How can they be going about their day, acting as if everything is normal?" I asked myself. But everything *was* normal as far as they knew.

This was the first of many times over the next months that my emotions shifted quickly and irrationally, a roller coaster ride in the theme park of cancer and cancer treatment.

Fortunately, the ride leveled out that morning, and, sobbing for the first time since the diagnosis, I told my parents. Three of my mother's four sisters were living with breast cancer, and she herself had been diagnosed with lymphoma five years earlier. She knew what was ahead for me, and what she and my dad could—and could not—do as I went through the difficult days.

They let me cry, they promised me support, and they gave me love and pot roast. So what if it's cancer? You gotta eat. They brought me back to a feeling of normalcy, something I needed more than I imagined.

In the immediate aftermath of the diagnosis of any illness that is sure to disrupt the status quo, there are many things to be done.

You double-check insurance, particularly when many of the people and places you'd choose for care might not be approved by the managed care company that seemed just fine when all you needed was an antibiotic for a sore throat.

You talk to your employer about absence from work—how much you have available, how (or even if) you'll be paid, and what the expectations will be for your performance when you're on the job during and after treatment.

Suddenly you realize that hours have gone by, then days, and much of the time you've spent relating to other people has been about illness.

For me, this was a very difficult time. My legacy from my family was strength—and my interpretation of that strength was that it was generally best accomplished in silence, uncomplaining and accepting of one's lot.

Of course, right off the bat, I started talking. And, to my unending amazement, it didn't take away from my strength.

Even before the diagnosis, when the lump in my breast appeared in all its ominous uncertainty, I had seen a breast concerns counselor, a psychiatric nurse who had shifted the focus of her practice following her own experience with cancer.

She encouraged me to ask the questions I needed to ask and to talk about what I needed—to her, my doctors, my friends and family. Obviously I would ask questions of her and of my doctors; they're paid professionals. But it was harder with family and friends.

I had to learn to talk about what I needed—and what I didn't need. To do that I had to give up trying to control the outcome, trying to be sure their needs were met, too.

It was time to take care of myself, and to surround myself with those who could accept my awareness of my needs.

Sometimes in the face of illness, we need solitude, and it is important for others to respect that. In illness or in health, I have always found that time alone spent quietly or contemplatively, reading, or simply being, is the way that I renew my strength.

And, in an even more practical vein, it's also a time to formulate questions—to make lists of things you want to ask your medical team, and things you want to ask (or tell) your family and friends.

As the days approaching surgery ticked by, I learned a lot in solitude that led me to community. One thing that I realized was that I wanted to be open with my coworkers about what was going on in my life. No, I didn't have to share every detail, and, yes, I know that they aren't a therapy group. But my fear was that people wouldn't want to talk to me about it, and I didn't want it to be a secret. I didn't want it to get wrapped up in shame or fear (my own or others').

So I decided I would be open from the beginning.

Three days after the diagnosis, I shared the information I had at that point about the coming months of treatment in a meeting of the people I had worked with for the past seven years. These are men and women with whom I had a connection forged by all of our life experiences, from the birth of children to the death of parents to office politics. While we rarely socialized outside the office, we had been there for each other.

So I knew they would be there for me as I said, "I don't know how I'm going to handle this. I don't know how well I'll cope. I don't know what I'll need, and I don't know if I can ask."

But what I found over the next few months was an understanding that often brought me—and sometimes them—to tears. A loaf of home-baked bread delivered not the week of chemotherapy, when I couldn't eat, but the week after, when I could nibble; it always came, right on schedule. I never asked for it, because I didn't know how much I needed it.

Ditto for macaroni and cheese and banana bread from two other friends, who knew it would provide a little more sustenance on the "good days," those last days between treatments when the worst of the last one was over, and the next assault on my body had not yet begun.

I found, too, even before surgery, that there is a process of saying good-bye to life as you've known it. Some of that is done privately, while some can be shared.

I realized before my mastectomy that I would like to have a photograph of my breast. That called for understanding from another person, a reaching out that leaves you very vulnerable. But when we bring our vulnerability into a community where we feel safe—in my case, the workplace was one of several—we further strengthen that community of support.

So a couple of nights before the mastectomy, a photographer at the newspaper where I work, a woman who has been a friend (although not in a social setting) took pictures of me shirtless. Hugh Hefner would not be interested, but that was not the idea. I don't know why I needed to document the existence of my left breast, except that it was part of the patchwork of my life, and I needed every scrap I could gather to keep me whole.

Too, I had to begin to come to terms with how my body would change, a hurdle that comes with many life-threatening illnesses as disease and treatment take a highly visible physical toll. There is at best, I think, a self-consciousness, and at worst a fear that we will be unacceptable in our ravaged bodies.

Not everyone might want to start with a photographer, but that worked for me. In my case, not only was she another woman, but her mother had been diagnosed with breast cancer just weeks before. She knew before I even got the words out what I was asking for.

And she, like many others in the months to come, accepted me just where I was in a single moment.

Some of them were part of the sisterhood of breast cancer—it was something they had experienced, or their mothers had, or their sisters had. With some, I shared common experiences, and with others, we could pinpoint almost nothing in our lives that was similar.

But we learned from our differences, and we supported each other with our varied experiences.

And one afternoon, when I felt I had nothing to give, when I saw my illness and my physical weakness as a drain on people around me, a woman in my office made a point to come over and speak to me. "Because you've been willing to let us see your pain, I know that when I face a crisis I won't have to start at the beginning," she said.

So it was that I learned that there were many pilgrims sharing my journey. I learned that receiving can be a gift to others, too, and that in every human relationship, no matter how brief or how enduring, there is always an ebb and flow, a giving and a getting.

It is not answers that are required; it is presence. When one of us speaks and the other one listens, it is community, and it is healing.

Karen

Before he left me because of my cancer, my fiancé became less and less hopeful about my recovery. It was not until the day he left that he was explicit about that fact, but I could read it in offhand remarks he made about the future in a completely different way and in the subtle changes in his behavior. Before my diagnosis, we talked about the future a lot, as most engaged couples do. We dreamed about the kind of church we would create together. We talked about children, where we wanted to live, whether we would have an indoor dog, what kind of retirement we would work toward. We even joked about the fact that he was seven years younger than me: this was a good thing, we decided, because on average, men die seven years earlier than women do. So we fantasized that we would die on the same day, in each other's arms.

After I was diagnosed, I wanted to be married in the church but without a civil license, so we would not be "officially" married and he would therefore not be responsible for my medical bills. He agreed with this at first, and I even talked to our minister about it, who said he would gladly perform such a service. But after my metastasis was diagnosed, and as time went on, my fiancé talked less and less about marriage. Instead, he would make some announcement about his plans after graduation—plans that clearly did not include me. He became more reluctant to touch me. Our sexual relationship dried up quickly. I put that down to my belief that I was physically repulsive, with one and a half breasts and no hair. I told myself he was afraid to hurt me physically. But we had been great cuddlers, and even that stopped. He went so far as to stop sitting on the couch next to me, and would take the armchair across the room.

I loved this man very much, and we had often talked about how lucky we were to have found what few people do: a soul mate. I was devastated the day he left, and it took me months upon months to recover emotionally. I might say I still have not recovered; I have not been able to allow myself to get involved with anyone else. The danger of pain is too great; my heart is too battered to risk more hurt.

And yet as horrible as his abandonment was, I do believe that in the long run, it was one of the best things that could have happened to me.

Spending every day around someone who thought I was going to die soon made it difficult to believe otherwise. I needed to keep company with people who could hope for me, and he was not able to do that. If attitude has any contribution to physical health—and I think it does—then he did me a favor by exiting my life. Even by myself, I was able to be more hopeful than I was when he was around.

The many cards and letters I got in the mail during my treatment were incredibly helpful to me. Some days I would look in my mailbox to discover ten cards. When I was first diagnosed, they were all full of hope and encouragement. After my cancer metastasized, though, things changed. Some people were able to continue their encouragement, but others gave up on me. I vividly remember a card from someone I did not know well but with whom I had attended seminary. The front of the card was done in airbrushed pastels. The printed sentiment said, "As you go into the light, know that my prayers are with you." This was, I realized, a "Gee, sorry you're dying" card. First, I was thunderstruck that such a thing even existed. I was also furious to have in my hand solid proof that someone thought I was on the way out, and anticipated that would happen soon. While the card was unusual, the sentiment was not.

So many people seemed to think it was their job to get me in the right frame of mind to die. I am sure that from their point of view, I was "in denial." I had to wonder why people assumed I never thought about the seriousness of my illness unless they forced it upon me. If I had the guts at the time, I would have told them that I thought about it constantly, that hope was one of the most tenuous things in my life. I have that kind of chutzpah now, but at the time I just called a mutual acquaintance and asked her to tell the card's sender never to contact me again.

I knew the statistics; my oncologist had always been impeccably honest with me. I knew how unlikely it was that I would live five more years. That was the given. What I nurtured, held on to, tried to feed, and protected, was my hope. Sometimes I could not even hope for myself and had to lean on the hope other people had for me. So when someone intruded on me and tried to make me face "reality," it frightened and angered me.

The funny thing was that the people who were most hopeful for me in those days were the medical folks. That may have had something to do with the fact that my oncologist had cancer himself. He had been given only a 1 percent chance of survival, and yet there he was. He was honest with me, but he did not take away my hope. He said, in fact, that my continued hope was one of the things he admired about me. So why was it so hard for other people simply to allow me to hope, let alone to encourage me in it?

I was struck by how little hope the ministers I knew had for me. Certainly it is unfashionable to believe in miracles these days, but if you cannot expect that from the clergy, then who can you expect it from? I told some of my pastor friends that I perceived God working in my life, and they became angry. One fellow minister listened to me talk about my belief that God had kept me from death so far and said, "Oh, that's bullshit."

I suspect part of the problem was that people assumed cancer means death, and immediate death at that. I guess it used to. I also think I reminded them of their own mortality, so on an unconscious level at least, it would have been easier for *them* if I were not around any longer. And finally, I guess they thought I was not acting like a cancer patient "should" act. I "should" have been sitting around, morose and waiting to die, perking up only slightly when one of my acquaintances swooped in to tell me just exactly how desperate my situation was.

I did discover, to my surprise, that I had real friends, and they were not the people I expected. I discovered something about people: The ones most capable of intimacy are not necessarily the ones who are able to stick by in tough times. I have had a lot of friends in my life who are as intense as I am, who can sit and dissect a conversation for hours, think deeply about the meaning of the universe, examine their own souls, and speak to the depths of mine. But they were often the ones, it turned out, who ran away most quickly.

Then on the other hand, I have friends who are not exactly what I would call deep. They enjoy life and do not spend a lot of time agonizing over the great questions of the cosmos. They are sensible people who are a little amused by my tendency toward introspection. But I look around me after four and a half years of cancer, and they are the ones who remain.

I have come to value different things in people than I used to. In the past, nothing made me salivate more than being around brilliant, creative people. Now the friends I cherish so much tend to be a little more ordinary, with old-fashioned Boy Scout values like fidelity, stamina, honor, and truth. They are good, decent people, and plain in many ways. But they stood by me while the shining stars burned out quickly.

I was also surprised to find that the most deeply religious people I knew were not necessarily the most faithful or sensitive. Because I am a minister, at the time I was diagnosed I knew lots of other ministers. Perhaps it was because my illness struck too close to home that so many of them ran away or were ready to write me off. Ministers are used to taking care of other people; we have to have a certain amount of distance to be able to be present with them in the midst of their crises. But the fact that I was like them, a minister, meant the distance between caregiver and care-receiver was suddenly gone.

I do have faithful friends who are ministers, just as I have faithful friends who are deep and intense. But I have even more who are laypeople and—odd as it seems to me—atheists, agnostics, and, as one friend insists on calling herself, heathens.

I am more leery now of the tortured geniuses I run into in the course of my days. I will certainly sit and have tea with them and spend some time thinking out in the far reaches of the galaxy. I am always ready to trade war stories with other ministers, too. But they are not my real friends. Give me good, decent, ordinary people any day. They are my community.

Once I knew which people I could trust, I had to learn how to receive from them. I have the same disease that most ministers do: the need to be needed. It is extremely difficult for me to let anyone do anything for me. My parents come from the Appalachian Mountains, and I was raised to be extremely independent, a quality necessary for life in those hardscrabble hills and hollows. It took me thirty years or so to learn that in the city, anyway, *interdependence* is a healthier way of life than either dependence or independence.

I had this in my head at a theoretical level, but I do not think I really got it, really understood it, until my cancer treatment. Then I had no choice about allowing others to help me. At the most basic level, I had to have someone drive me to and from chemotherapy treatments; the pre-medications they gave me made me very sleepy and a danger on the road. My neediness only grew from there.

I found myself unbelievably weak from treatment. I finally discovered I could do two things a day, and those "things" included going to the grocery store, doing the laundry, or having lunch with someone. Before, between, and after those activities, I had to rest. That left a lot of very practical things undone in my life, and people came forward to help me. Thank God they did; despite all my protests, I could not have survived treatment without them.

The area in which I was raised to be most independent was with financial matters. From the age of seventeen, I pretty much made my own way. But cancer treatment meant I could not work, and while I had a scholarship to cover tuition, I still had to pay rent, buy groceries, and meet my medical bills. I was deeply moved when a dear woman in my congregation asked if it was all right for a group of people to hold a fund-raiser for me. It was hard to say "Yes," but I really and truly had no choice. I needed the money. Even if it was only $200, I needed the money. So on the night of the talent show and barbecue dinner that made up the fund-raising event, I wept when they called me up to give me the check. When they announced it was for more than $4,000, I absolutely sobbed. Never before in my life had anyone been so generous to me.

People helped me in tiny ways, too, that were very important. The day my temperature skyrocketed to 104 degrees and I had to be admitted to the hospital through the emergency room, I was miserably sick and frightened as well. The X ray technician came in to take me for a chest film, and the whole time he was with me he kept up a soft, soothing patter, telling me what he was doing, how much longer it was going to be, and what would happen next. That man, whose name I never knew, made that whole experience bearable for me.

I got to know the manager at the wig store pretty well. I had no idea, when I bought my first wig, that I would need one for a year and a half and that wigs wear out. She did not turn away a bit when she saw my bald head, and she spent a great deal of time trying to find the right style for me. She had alopecia, and shared many tips on how to live without hair. When I finally got off chemotherapy, I went by the store to show her my inch-long hair. She jumped up and down, even though it meant I would not be spending money at her store anymore.

I have never really reflected before on the qualities that separated the helpful people in my life from the harmful ones. I think it has much to do with their ability to take me as I am, even if they do not agree with my theology or despite the fact that my talk of death frightens them. They all seem to have the ability to listen, and listen a long time, without having to interrupt and offer whatever "solution" they can think of. Most important to me, though, is loyalty. When I meet new people these days, I always ask myself, "Will they stick by me when it gets bad again?" Sometimes the answer is "Yes," and I treasure those new friends as much as I do the veterans. Sometimes the answer is "No," and while I still interact with those people, I simply do not invest in them very deeply.

Before I had cancer, the thought that I would have to "protect" myself from anyone besides physically violent people was completely foreign to me. I have learned the hard way that the most gentle-seeming people can do me incredible harm. While I may be angry at the ways these folks have treated me, I cannot say I condemn them. They simply do not have it in them to be a friend to a cancer patient. I feel sorry for them, in a way. I think they live in fear. I am afraid, too, but I get out of bed and live my life despite my fear of illness and death. By isolating themselves from me, whether by abandonment or stupidity, these people show that they are ruled by fear. In avoiding me, they hope to avoid death; in fact, they are avoiding life. I must protect myself from them, but I pity them perhaps even more.

Susan

> "From you I receive, to you I give, together we share,
> from this we live."
These words from Rabbi Hillel have been put to music.
We sing them in our Universal Worship service, an

activity of my meditation school. We celebrate the major
world religions with Scripture, music, and dance. Did
Hillel mean "You" as is in God or "you" as in people?
Is this not the essence of religion, that the love of
God is our love for one another?

❧

A sweet dance goes with the song. Partners face each
other and form a circle. They make gestures of receiving
and giving. On the "together we share" phrase,
each places a hand gently on the partner's heart. During
the last phrase, the partners bow to each other,
in love and respect. Then one partner advances,
and the dance repeats itself.
The remarkable part of this dance is noticing the
unique gift of each person as he or she stands
before you, and then moves on.

There are many ways to heal from cancer. Healing does not necessarily
mean surviving, for, as my surgeon says, "Life is a lethal condition."
Healing is about learning to live. Healing the body through medical
treatment is only the beginning. The next part of healing comes when
we piece our lives back together, and reconnect the threads that were severed by illness. This is the stage of community. The questions of community are these: How do find our place again? How do we give? How
do we receive? How can we be there for one another?

This stage of healing goes beyond the realm of medical institutions,
although many sponsor supporting activities. We are all part of this
community of healing. How much a part are we willing to play?

With all the awareness and education about cancer, I assumed that
people who are ill find communities of support. This is not always true.
My brother-in-law, John, died of a brain tumor this year. He was fifty
years old. Experimental chemotherapy allowed him to live almost two
years past diagnosis. The family stayed close during this time. My sister
was able to meet her promise that she would care for him, that he would
keep his dignity, and that the family would surround him with love.

John was a tender man and a devoted husband and father. He was also a high-powered Washington, D.C. lawyer, an extraordinary litigator. He had a long roster of prominent physicians and civic leaders whom he saved from nasty lawsuits. As his disease progressed, John's body became bloated from the steroids, his speech was confused, and he could no longer drive his car. He was often at home alone. He passed the time making model airplanes. By the time he died, over thirty brightly colored planes hung from the ceiling of the family room.

On the day of John's funeral, I sat with many visitors. I look exactly like my sister and they thought they were talking to her. One after the other they said, "I had been meaning to visit." "I didn't know he was so sick." "He was a fabulous lawyer. If it weren't for him I..." Even the rabbi said he had been meaning to call. They wanted absolution from me, to tell them it was not their fault, that they were busy, that they meant well. I did not have to say a thing. As they spoke, I could see the remorse in their eyes.

I asked my sister for one of the airplanes. Three months after John's death, my sister came to Nashville for my graduation. I had earned my doctorate in education after eight years in graduate school. This was a real celebration, since my cancer diagnosis came in the middle of my studies. My sister presented me with a large box. Inside was an airplane, a bright, yellow World War II model with red markings. A tiny pilot sat in the cockpit. Fragile spindles held the wheels.

I keep this airplane on a prominent shelf in our living room. When people notice it, many suggest that it symbolizes my soaring through troubles to a new horizon. This is not what it means to me. I love the airplane, not because it flies, because it couldn't possibly. It is decrepit. The wheels fall off every time I move it. The pilot falls out of his seat. I had to reglue the propeller. It stuck, but it no longer turns.

What does the airplane mean to me? The airplane is a promise to myself to notice those who are suffering, people who are ill, and their families who bear the indescribably difficult task of daily caretaking. To visit, to phone, to take food, a book, or to run an errand. In this enlightened age of information, when it is not shameful to speak of illness, one would think that communities would gather around someone with cancer. Sadly, there are many like my brother-in-law, who suffer not only with the disease but with loneliness and isolation. I think of the line of the Shaker song, "If we love not one another in daily communion, how can we love God who we have not seen?" My meditation practice helps me remember God. The airplane reminds me how to love others.

Are there people from whom we should not receive? Absolutely. Carol has been reading the advice books for people with cancer. One famous physician explained his system of coping by drawing pictures about your illness. This author goes on to give what he considers to be the correct system of interpretation. If the drawing is purple, it means you have a death wish.

Carol and I went to a workshop where we were asked to make a drawing. We were given a box of colored markers. Carol drew vibrant gold fish. But she avoided the purple marker. She was remembering the advice of this author, and did not want to wish herself dead. Walking out the door, we questioned this doctor's interpretive system. Who was he to say what our drawings meant?

The next week, Carol made another drawing. This time it was of a giant goldfish with huge purple eyes. She explained she needed to use the purple to not be afraid of it anymore. To her, the purple eyes in the fish mean "I have seen death, and while it changed me, I am alive."

The drawing makes her happy, for it is coming from the truth of her experience. There are many experts out there, waiting to tell us what our cancer means. Take their advice with a grain of salt. No one can interpret another's illness. Meaning unfolds in its own time, in its own way. The richness is in finding the unique meaning for ourselves. What we discover becomes a gift to those who hear our stories.

Whatever comes next, I will face it both alone and with others. So will Carol. And Karen. And Linda. And the million people in the United States who will be diagnosed with cancer this year. Five hundred thousand will die. Even when the cure for cancer is found, there will always be suffering.

There is a famous story about the Buddha. A woman came to him, distraught with her troubles. He told her she would be healed if she could obtain a mustard seed from a household where no one had suffered. The woman tried to find such a family. At each door, she heard accounts of sadness and grief. These encounters opened her heart and with that understanding, she was healed.

What did she learn? Perhaps a story from the Jewish tradition holds something of the answer. It is said that God made the world as a perfect clay vessel. God entrusted one of her Chief Angels to deliver it. On the way, the angel tripped. The clay vessel broke and was shattered into billions of pieces. Rather than leaving us in a world that was already perfect, God left us with much work to do. In Hebrew, this work is called *Tikkun Olam.* It means "the restoration of the world," knitting the pieces back together. We do this by regarding one another and gathering together in communities bound by love. We cannot stop suffering, prevent illness, or overcome death. But there are things we can do.

We can stand by. We can be witnesses. We can listen. We can offer support. We can advocate for better treatment and more awareness. We can reach out to those who are suffering alone. We can help one another find our own stories, for each of us has wisdom to convey. Sometimes, the things we do for one another may not seem like much. We notice the heroics of a medical procedure, but many more miracles happen far away from the limelight.

My husband, rather than turning away in disgust at my mastectomy, got out his sculpture materials and made me a breast. Carol sat on my bed while I was recovering from one of several surgeries. I cannot remember what we said, but I remember her presence. My sister called every day. There are hundreds of such gestures that wrap around me, a true gift from a community of people who care. It was surprising who these people turned out to be. Most who came forward were those well acquainted with suffering. The gestures came from their hearts. Others, who I expected to support me, seemed to fade away. I developed a meter that detected genuineness. I lost my tolerance for artifice. Like a wild animal who knows which grasses to eat, I was attracted to those whose presence brought healing, and repelled by those whose did not. These signals were not subtle, but very clear, like a light that was green or red. I learned to heed them. I have heard from others with cancer who share this same discovery.

If I learned anything at all from cancer, it is that there are hundreds of loving hearts within reach. I found them where I least expected them.

I found them among friends, and in the medical center. I also learned that many people turn away from those who are ill, for whatever reason. Perhaps it is because of discomfort, fear of death, not knowing what to say, or simply being too busy. It is true that we cannot stop suffering. But we can remember the lesson of *Tikkun Olam*. We can knit the world together.

Cancer takes us into a treacherous terrain where we need the interventions and counsel of experts. But the best gifts are the most ordinary, the simple gestures of kindness and concern. We also give gifts by telling our stories, for when they are genuine, they become stepping stones for those who inevitably follow on this path.

Spirit

THIS IS THE STAGE OF INTEGRATION, of looking back and at the same time looking forward. How can I find peace of mind when I'm living my life over the edge? What have I learned? This is the time when we digest the intense experiences that have come before, and in so doing find inner strength, hope, and, most of all, appreciation for the sacredness of life. Whatever happens in life is our spiritual path. With this wisdom, we can gently guide others through this terrain. What can others do at this time? Listen and learn from us.

Wheresoever you go, go with all your heart.
—CONFUCIUS

When a woman is diagnosed with breast cancer, she has the opportunity to confront the unknown future and the precious present. Even the most spiritual among us must learn to live in the shadow of uncertainty. But given the fact that we all must die someday—coupled with the volatility of life today, with drive-by shootings, carjackings, home invasions, plummeting jets, and natural disasters—this may not be such an unfortunate skill to have to master.

On this journey, it is possible to learn not only to live with that uncertainty, but to move through it with something that approaches grace.

Spiritual teaching is there for the asking for those who face life-threatening illness. It is an experience that offers ongoing dialogue in response to the questions that are central to spiritual growth: What have we learned about the meaning of our own lives in particular, and life in general? How do we relate to our lives differently than before? What has this experience been—and what does it continue to be—about?

And so the journey continues.

EIGHT

How Can I Find Peace of Mind When I'm Living My Life Over the Edge?

Carol

You may remember the story from the Buddhist tradition that Susan told earlier, in which a grieving woman goes to every house in the village, looking for a family that has not seen sorrow. She cannot find a single house that has not been touched. She returns to the Buddha to tell of her failure and instantly attains enlightenment.

I thought of this story many times the day after my diagnosis. Numb with the weight of my breast cancer, one of my first thoughts was to touch base with my everyday community, my fellow students, the administrators and teachers at Vanderbilt Divinity School. As I entered the familiar hallways of my school, I felt like a ghost—already dead. Since it was near the end of the semester, many of my classmates were buried under books at the library or shuffling reams of paper in their apartments and rooms. The school was unnaturally quiet. But I urgently I felt the need to tap even momentarily into the everyday reality that just yesterday had so neatly defined a large portion of my life.

I rounded the first corner, heading toward the common room, and spotted the teaching assistant for my ethics class, an attractive woman in her late twenties. Quietly, I took her aside and told her my news. She looked aghast. Then, she shared with me something very few people knew: her mother had breast cancer. She'd had a mastectomy and radiation and five years later was doing fine. She confessed to me that knew that her own odds were higher than the population at large, and secretly struggled with her fear. It was something she was learning to live with. She gave me a big hug and told me to call on her for anything, any time. I thanked her for her support and walked on. In the common room, I came upon two of my classmates. "Where were you yesterday?" they asked. I told them my sad story. The first of my friends responded, "You too? I had a malignant lump removed several years ago. In fact, the cancer was instrumental in my decision to come to divinity school." The second of my friends then volunteered that even as we stood there together, she was waiting to go see her doctor that afternoon, having had a worrisome Pap smear. With more hugs and prayers, I headed for the office of one of the divinity school's administrators.

"Carol, do you remember that right after you started school I disappeared for awhile? What I was doing was undergoing surgery and chemotherapy for breast cancer."

"You were? But you didn't say anything!"

"I kept it very quiet. Only a few people knew."

On that first day back to school after my diagnosis, I encountered seven women walking down hallways, hanging out in the bookstore, working in their offices. Of the seven, every single one of them either had cancer (or something equally serious) in their past or present, or had a parent or sister or close friend who had. Rather than feel sorry for myself, by the end of that day, I felt humbled and awestruck by the grace and dignity of a whole new world that was opening up to me. I felt privileged to be let in so deeply into my friends' and associates' secret inner lives. I lost the brash innocence of youth, but I gained access to the richness of courage, strength, and faith that lies hidden beneath the surface of so many of our everyday lives. The truth is, I realized, that we are all living our lives over the edge—it's just that some of us know it, and some of us do not.

I vowed to emulate my friends' courage as the following critical days and weeks unfolded in my life. When I pulled a back muscle, complaining of the sudden onslaught of lower back pain, the doctor felt compelled to send me for a bone scan. Lying alone on a cold metal slab, a huge whirring machine scanning my body for cancer, I was the most afraid I've ever been. What scared me as much as the machines were the technicians, who treated me as if I were a subject rather than a person. This hospital is a training facility. I could hear every word the senior technician was sharing with her associate. "See here, this is the hip joint." She went on to describe the various attributes of the bones, organs, and tissues they were encountering on the scanner screen in detail. Oh, my God. I didn't want to overhear them casually remarking on something abnormal in the scan. This was not how I wanted to learn if my cancer had metastasized.

To handle the fear, and drown out their conversation, I began to sing. I sang songs from every Broadway musical I could remember. Loud. And when the scan still had not ended, I started in on campfire spirituals. You've never seen anybody get up, get dressed, and get out of a treatment facility as fast as did I on that day. When my doctor gave me the results later that afternoon, the news was good. But just as important, it was delivered to me on my own terms, in a time, place, and way that respected my needs.

Taking care of myself did not come naturally. I had to learn how to take control over whatever I could: I soon learned not to be ashamed of asking for my favorite nurse, even if I hurt the student nurse's feelings, or an extra blanket, even if it meant someone had to go to the other end of the house to fetch it. If I needed pain medication, or something to cut my anxiety, I got it. This was no time for self-sacrifice or martyrdom.

At the same time, I had to make sure I was being taken care of spiritually. The story of Jacob struggling on the banks of the Jabbok River came often to mind. In this story from the Hebrew Scriptures, Jacob, son of Isaac, was ever-seeking to win God's blessing—but his efforts were flawed. He cheated his brother Esau of his birthright, then left home to make his fortune. Despite his riches, his many wives and children, he was not at peace. And so it was that he decided to journey to his childhood home with his entourage, traveling many days and nights. When the caravan reached the banks of the Jabbok, their last resting place before arriving at his destination, Jacob sent the others on ahead. Alone in the dark, he was visited by an agent of God. Jacob and the angel embarked upon a life and death struggle. All night long, they wrestled on the banks of the Jabbok. Exhausted, still Jacob would not stop wrestling until he won God's blessing. When morning dawned, wounded and limping, Jacob at last received what he came for. Jacob had been willing to take a stand for what he wanted—to put his very life on the line for it. And in the end, he got what he wanted.

I identified with Jacob, feeling that physically and spiritually, I was also wrestling through the dark night in order to wrest free God's blessing.

Toward the end of chemotherapy, I suddenly became feverish and weepy. Dan came to sit by my side, wiping my brow.

"What is it?" he asked, concerned.

"Dan, I knew there was something important about undergoing seven rounds of chemotherapy. It felt like a ritual purification—a spiritual cleansing. I feel like I've walked through fire to get here, and now it's nearly over."

"Then why are you crying?" he asked.

"Because I always thought I would emerge from this whole and into something specific. You know, I would be more advanced spiritually. Or my writing would be more profound. Or I would have some guarantee that the cancer will never come back. Something tangible that I could put my hands on. But it's not like that at all. I know now that I'm emerging whole—and into emptiness. I don't know what the future will bring."

"No wonder you're crying! It sounds really scary!"

"No, you don't understand! I'm crying because I'm so afraid I'll forget this feeling of absolute freedom. It feels like anything is possible and everything's all right."

I understand why in some Eastern religions, it is considered to be a
high spiritual practice to meditate in a graveyard. Confronting mortality puts our everyday stresses and strains—and even our extraordinary
ones—into broader perspective. As the days turn into months since my
last treatment, I pause to remember what it felt like during those seven
rounds to have so very little separating my heart from the divine. To be
in unity with God is an ultimate state, in and of itself. Serving God in
this way is something one can do sick or well. It is a foretaste of what lies
ahead for us all.

After I finished chemotherapy, I was excited about reentering the
mainstream of my life. It was as if I'd been shot from a cannon, there was
so much I wanted to accomplish! There was one problem, however.
Every afternoon, around 3 or 4 P.M., I'd be absolutely exhausted. Em
told me I needed to rest. I fought the idea, but eventually I surrendered.
I finally convinced myself to take daily naps, telling myself, "I need to
rest so that I don't get cancer again." This worked, in that it got me to
lie down in the middle of the day, but more often than not, the concern
about the possible recurrence of cancer made my naps fitful at best. I
went to see Em.

"Stop reinforcing your fears," she advised. "When you need to give
yourself a break, don't tell yourself it's to prevent a recurrence. Instead,
tell yourself that you need to rest because you're tired. You are the kind
of person who takes good care of herself, who instinctively knows what
she needs to do to support her healing."

I am reminded of a favorite quote from the *I Ching*, the ancient
Chinese book of wisdom that had inspired a number of my early books.
To paraphrase: "When a strong woman meets with adversity, she
remains cheerful despite all danger, and this cheerfulness is the source of
later successes. It is this stability which is stronger than fate. If adversity
only bends a woman, it creates in her a power to react that in time will
manifest itself."

Admittedly, I am not cheerful all the time. Sometimes I'm cranky,
sometimes I'm angry or fearful or depressed. But I have learned that if I
hold my emotions lightly, they change. Feelings are like the weather. It's
sunny one day, stormy the next. You don't need to do anything to make
the sun shine sooner or later, and you don't need to do anything to make

the fear pass. If you can't be cheerful in the midst of the storm, you can at least have the kind of stability that comes when you stop trying to hold onto this or that mood and instead expand your willingness to embrace it all.

Susan

Cancer taught me how to live life over the edge. In the language of the mystics, this is awakening. Most people go through their lives asleep. We anesthetize ourselves with drugs, alcohol, television, or the flickering of a computer screen. We busy ourselves with incessant work and constant activity.

People pay thousands of dollars to enjoy life more. We have massages, facials, and mud baths. We attend workshops on psychology, meditation, swimming with dolphins, drumming, journaling, climbing ropes, ancient teachings—the list goes on. We can find our inner child, our tribal mind, our lost soul, our past life, or our spirit guide. I admit it, I go to some of these myself. However, nothing had the same effect on my consciousness as my experience with cancer.

I went to visit Carol in the hospital while she was recovering from her mastectomy. Her friends from divinity school who came to make a call on the infirm may have been a tad disappointed. She looked radiant. "You know," she said, "this is like a spa and a spiritual retreat rolled into one." We laughed uproariously as we had done many times while comparing our cancer tales. We knew we were being propelled over the edge. And we were thrilled.

I am so fortunate. Yes, I have cancer, but I have been given the opportunity to live and learn extraordinary things. Others who face cancer agree. As a friend said, "Now, I like to sit around and watch the grass grow." Life is such a miracle.

One of the questions I keep wondering is, "Would I have come to this realization without cancer?" I cannot say, but this is one of the reasons I want to share what I have learned. I am trying to pinpoint just what it is about cancer that is jet fuel to my spirit. I want to understand it, distill it, and make it available to others. Surely, one can learn this without having cancer. My quest is to find out how.

Do I have peace of mind? If peace of mind means being tranquil, I would say, "No." I worry. I fret. I am intensely expressive and passionate, as if an invisible set of personality brakes was removed. I no longer worry much about what people think of me. I have a set of problems completely unrelated to cancer. My mind is not at peace. But I am content. I want to succeed at what I do, but I have little ambition for status or power. I have all the power I need. I am beginning to understand what is meant by the power of love and the force of life.

I am determined to live what I have learned. Some people's response to cancer is to get back to routine, to work, and to forget. I want to remember. Six months after my treatment ended, when my normal energy returned, I made a promise to myself. I wrote this in my journal:

ESSENTIALS

I am back at work now and feel the driving rhythm of my responsibilities trying to draw me into an automatic state, rushing from crisis to crisis. I am afraid my work, though I love it, will tarnish the precious gift I have discovered in my life. This is such an old story, of the one who recovers from cancer, who gets to come back into life. I can still feel a sweet sensitivity, opened somehow in the process of illness and healing. I never want to lose it.

This experience, all of it, has changed the ground of my being, the tone of my emotions, the tenor of my mind, and the texture of my heart. I suppose each person must discover her own list of essentials. Here are some of mine. I am practicing how to say them precisely, for they are as lovely, perfect, and unique as flowers or gems. I am still revising.

Be tender to the ones who love me.

Spend more time with family and friends.

Hang out with lots of children.

Stick to what is real.

Act with courage.

Stand on the ground of simplicity.

Be vigilant. Guard my opened eyes. Do not doubt their vision.

Care for the people who come my way.

Hold in my heart those whose call.

Cherish this precious gift of life.

Karen

"I worry about you in that car," said a friend to me recently. "It's a death trap." It is, actually. It's a subcompact car and the metal is very thin. I won't name the maker because there is no reason to embarrass them when there are so many other cars like it. When I bought it seven years ago, I chose it because of the sticker price, nothing more and nothing less. But I answered my friend, "Not a bad way to go though, all at once."

As the member of the cancer initiates and as a pastor, I have had all too many chances to be with someone while he or she dies. Most of my cancer friends who die follow a certain pattern. As long as they can stay up and around, they do. Once they take to their beds, though, they go pretty fast. One exception was my friend Carolyn. She came to our support group soon after her surgery for ovarian cancer and she had already started her chemotherapy. She lived much longer than anyone predicted, and during those years she had over a hundred chemotherapy treatments. There came the point when Carolyn had to go into the hospital. Some of us from support group went to visit her and say good-bye. "I'll see you in the good place," I told her, and left, expecting to get a phone call any day that she had died. But it took her weeks to finally go. Maybe she had gotten so deeply entrenched in the habit of fighting to live that she just could not stop. Those were miserable weeks: painful for her, agonizing for her son and father, a horror for her friends.

As a pastor, I also get to see the aftermath of someone's death. I have discovered some truths about dying. One is that while a sudden, quick death is more difficult for the survivors, a long, lingering death is harder for the one who dies.

I hope and pray, quite literally, that when my time comes, it will be fast. I have a living will stating I do not want extraordinary means used to prolong my life. But I have heard horror stories of people who are rushed into the emergency room clinically dead, and are shocked back into life. It is only after they are stable that the chart arrives and its first page is a living will and, in the parlance of the medical world, a "DNR." Do Not Resuscitate. That scenario is one that gives me nightmares. I have even considered having "DNR" tattooed on my chest, between my breasts.

As I write, I can hear the voices of my healthy friends quite vividly: "Karen, that's so morbid!" I guess in one way it is, because I have been pondering the way in which I hope to die. But I could reply to my friends that it is not morbid; in fact, it is simply realistic.

One of the hard truths of life is that it ends for each of us. I have said it before and I will say it again: In America, we try to forget that fact; we try to pretend it is not true; we do everything we can to postpone it. Having traveled the road I have, I must say I think we have it completely backward.

It is the very transience of life that makes it precious. If we all expected to live forever, life would not amount to much. It would become very cheap. In fact, I suspect this is just what has happened in our culture. We have convinced ourselves, as a society, that death does not exist. We are in denial, as Ernst Becker tells us. It is only because life is so cheap that we have horrifying modern realities like five-year-old children committing murder. It is only because we regard life so little that we allow children to be the majority of the poor people in this country. I sometimes think that the United States went from barbarism to decadence without a period of civilization in between.

But this philosophical/theological matter is not the question here. I should be speaking much more practically: Given the reality of death, how do I find peace of mind? I have been forced into many of the suggestions that follow, but I wish I had been able to learn about them without a cancer diagnosis.

The first and most important thing I had to do to live peacefully was to stop denying my death. Cancer forced that on me. Even when I was first diagnosed and going through what I hoped would be my only treatment, I was struck by a surprising new thought: "Even if the cancer doesn't get me, something will. And it could happen any time." There are ways to learn this and believe it without having a terrible physical diagnosis.

It is a very good exercise to plan one's own funeral. There are two parts to that process, and I heartily recommend both to everyone. The first is going to the funeral home. Not only is this a good spiritual discipline, it is also a great kindness to the people we will leave behind. The funeral industry preys on the guilt that so often accompanies someone's death, and our relatives very well may end up spending a ridiculous amount of money on our funerals when we would not want that sacrifice from them. If we make arrangements with the funeral home ourselves, then we can spare the people we love.

Here is an odd thought: One of the selling points for caskets is how leakproof they are. The longer the casket will keep out water and worms, the more it costs. Why in the world would anyone pay thousands of dollars for such a thing? I do not know of any religious system since the Egyptians that believes we will need these bodies in the afterlife. The fact is that a dead body will decay—as it is supposed to—whether it is buried in an $8,000 guaranteed-leakproof-for-two-hundred-years casket or in a simple pine box. Choosing our own casket can make it clear to us how fragile, impermanent, and organic our bodies are.

The second part of arranging one's own funeral is the religious service, if you want one. Even people who are not religious usually have some sort of memorial, and it makes sense to have that service reflect who we were in life. There is nothing I detest more than the warbly organ music I find in most Southern funeral homes, so in the funeral I have planned, I have named the music I want played before the funeral begins: "Cantus in Memory of Benjamin Britten" by Arvo Part; "Adagio for Strings" by Samuel Barber; and the "Sarabande" from Bach's *Cello Suite no. 2 in D Minor*. I want people to leave the service to the accompaniment of Arcangelo Corelli's *Concerto Grosso, Opus 6, no. 8* and "It is Accomplished" from Peter Gabriel's *Passion*. As a minister, I have always insisted on as much congregational participation as possible, so I do not want people just sitting there as if they are spectators at a performance. I want them all to sing "Be Thou My Vision." And I want my friend Ami Faenza to use her gorgeous voice to sing, "I Will Rise and Go to Jesus." The point I am making is not to tell the world what kind of funeral music I want, but that it is necessary to get to this level of detail in order to come out of denial about our deaths.

Another important activity is writing a will. Many people have substantial assets that they have to take care of, and so they turn the will over to a lawyer—and usually forget about it. But whether we have millions of dollars or very little, the spiritually important part of a will is not disposing of our "valuable" things, as our culture counts them, but of the things that have a place in our hearts. When I worked on my will, I went through my home and listed everything I owned that had sentimental value, and I decided whom I wanted each to go to. I have not decided, if I have notice of my death, whether to let those things go to my friends after I die, or whether to give them away while I am still living with an explanation of what the gifts mean.

Getting over our denial of death is a constant process. Even I, The Terminal One, fall back into denial on occasion. Given my situation, something usually reminds me, even if it is nothing more than my monthly treatment. Folks who are simply terminal in the way all of us are will probably have to be more intentional about staying aware of death.

It sounds odd to say, but I believe that a true awareness of death gives us most of what we need to deal with its reality. Along with that awareness come the wide-open eyes I mentioned before, a pressing need to decide what we believe about life after death, and eventually, a sense of peace.

The fact is that we all live "over the edge," and it is counterintuitive to imagine that peace can come out of living in awareness of that reality. But I am reminded, once again, of my dancing skeleton stamp. Knowing that I will die—perhaps in a year or two, perhaps this afternoon—is exactly what makes me savor life. I have stopped fighting awareness of one of the most important aspects of my existence, and after that struggle was over, I found peace at the center of my soul. The way to live over the edge with peace is simply to go ahead and face the truth.

Linda

The wheel is always turning, Joseph Campbell tells us. To center ourselves, we must live at the center, rather than lashed to the spokes. In the best of times, when we are close to our higher power, when we are listening to our inner voice, the center is still a difficult place to reach, to settle into.

Ironically, it is more accessible in the dark night of the soul, and when life-threatening illness enters our lives, it is the place we strive to come to.

I had been a seeker, long before cancer, but no matter how hard I tried, I couldn't find the center. Days of my life passed while I was holding on to the wheel as it spun ever faster, then stopped abruptly, switched directions, and lurched forward.

The prevalent image in my mind was of a cruel, heavy-booted Nazi pushing quarter after quarter into the ticket booth at what was for no good reason called an amusement park. High above him, desperately hanging on to the wheel, I could only watch. And wait.

That is the way I had lived, anxiety rising, then numbed with alcohol. I could not imagine how I could ever do it any other way. Eventually, however, I did, through a recovery program that introduced me not only to abstinence but also to acceptance. I've worked that program for thirteen years.

By the time cancer arrived, acceptance was no longer a foreign concept. During those days and months that extended to years, I tried to view illness not as catastrophe, but as possibility. All I can tell you is that sometimes it worked.

But when I became aware that the end of cancer treatment was not the end of the illness, that life would not revert to P.C.—pre-cancer—status, it was hard not to feel overwhelmed.

There's an entry on my calendar on December 20, 1993, the last day of my treatment for breast cancer, that's brief and to the point: "Radiation. The End."

Well, not quite.

During treatment, I had ignored my reconstruction, a misshapen mass of abdominal tissue that just a few weeks after surgery had balked at becoming my left breast.

A year after the mastectomy and initial reconstruction, we tried again, this time using the latissimus dorsi muscle, which was channeled from my back, below my shoulder blade, to the area where the earlier tissue loss had left a sunken scar.

So far, so good. My hair had grown back since the end of chemotherapy, and I got a mini-haircut two months later. Now I had breasts that were beginning to match if you kind of squinted when you looked at them. The fatigue was still extraordinary, but I was aware that I was very gradually getting stronger. The catheter by which chemotherapy had been administered had been removed from my chest in a minor surgical procedure, and a few months later my horror at discovering a new breast lump turned to relief after it was removed and determined to be benign.

I was amazed at how quickly I forgot about it. Life was getting back to normal.

Then I began a series of setbacks with the reconstruction that no one could have predicted, that left a team of fine plastic surgeons scratching their heads. Three more surgeries and even more scars followed. When it became evident that there would be yet another surgery, I really struggled with whether or not I wanted to continue. Maybe my body was trying to tell me that I didn't need to cover up the tumor site. With each surgery and the added scar tissue, it became more and more difficult to determine what was "normal," that is, what lumps and knots had been created by surgery and which, if any, might be cancer-related.

So, I made a decision. Three weeks after what I expected to be my last reconstructive surgery, I put on a very snug sports bra to hold my breasts/chest in place, and I went hiking in Mexico. For me, it was time to say, "Enough. For whatever days I have, I will live." That was the beginning of my real recovery, my effort to put breast cancer in some permanent perspective in my life, to acknowledge its significance, but to subdue its enormity.

Serendipitously, on that trip to the Copper Canyon of Mexico, I met a classical pianist, Romayne Wheeler, who lives most of the year among the Tarahumara Indians. They call themselves "the light-footed ones," and are known for running long distances without stopping.

That would not be the lesson I would learn from them, since even slow hiking was physically difficult for me at the time. Rather, I had the opportunity to learn about some of their basic beliefs, particularly that a thing is rarely judged to be bad or good. Instead, the Tarahumara "say something serves life or something doesn't serve life," Wheeler wrote in *Life through the Eyes of a Tarahumara*.

The Indians believe that worry and despair do not serve life. "Cleanse your life from anxiety, from impatience, from so many things that string you up-tight and separate you from Our Mother the Earth. Then you will find tranquility," Wheeler wrote.

It helped me to better understand that a life on the edge—in my case, driven there by cancer—not only could not foster peace, it could not even accommodate it.

Since then, I have tried, at a deep but conscious level, to stay at the center of the wheel Joseph Campbell described. There are times when it is perched precariously close to some ledge or other, some place where a blood test or a bone scan might tip the balance. The impulse then is to grab a spoke and hold on, but if the wheel keeps on turning—and that is the business of a wheel—it is inevitable that I will be pulled from the center, perhaps wrenched from the wheel and hurled into chaos once more. Given my experience with cancer, I would say that it is even likely.

Knowing that and still maintaining something that resembles peace of mind are difficult to reconcile, but neither is exclusive of the other. In illness, I sometimes considered present and future, and felt that all would be won or all would be lost. But that would be too easy.

If we choose consciousness, if we keep ourselves open to awareness, then we are carried from darkness to light, from joy to despair, carried there and then brought back again. It is in the repetition that we learn. It is when our expectations are unfulfilled, and our semblance of well-ordered lives is disrupted that we can search our souls—if we've found them, of course.

"Life is neither ordered nor disordered; life just is," Christina Baldwin wrote in *Life's Companion*. "Disorder comes through the process of having our assumptions challenged, sometimes brutally challenged. In the gap, we learn to re-perceive life, to review our assumptions, to adjust to altered conditions for travel." In short, we can find what anguish has to offer. All in all, it has far greater potential than joy. Ultimately, we are clearing our own spiritual path into directions that have not yet been revealed to us. If we do it honestly, we will find our way, even though we don't know what it is at the outset.

William Least Heat Moon, writer, traveler, and professor, made a literal journey that in many ways was parallel to a spiritual one. When Least Heat Moon stopped one morning in a town in Tennessee, as he writes in *Blue Highways,* the storekeeper made conversation while filling Least Heat Moon's car with gasoline.

"Where you going?" the storekeeper asked.

"Don't know," the traveler replied.

"Well, you can't get lost then," the storekeeper concluded.

NINE

What Have I Learned?

Linda

In T. H. White's wonderful book, *The Once and Future King,* which took him twenty-five years to write—a good example of keeping on keeping on, no matter what—he wrote, "'The best thing for being sad,' replied Merlin, beginning to puff and blow, 'is to learn something. That is the only thing that never fails.'"

And so in long, lonely, predawn hours, I tried to embrace the lessons of an illness that threatened life as I'd known it. I asked myself, "If you cannot learn from this, what can you learn from?"

So I learned to let people love me; I learned to ask for help; and I learned that the real measure of my healing would not be about a cure in my body. No, healing would happen in my heart and soul. I would be at peace.

But, of course, I had to learn to recognize it when it arrived, and that is perhaps the greatest lesson of all.

When your life is threatened and someone promises a cure, it is instinctive to embrace that. In doing that, however, it is easy to overlook the greater gift that is being offered.

There is a story in Christian tradition in which Jesus performs what the people perceive to be miracles—a leper is healed of his sores, a deaf man hears. The joy and amazement expressed by those who witness these events focus on the physical cures they have seen, but the miracle worker is offering a greater lesson that can be found in quiet contemplation—the peace of the kingdom of God.

In the twelve-step tradition, which borrows a great deal from Christianity, there is that same promise. No matter the depths of our suffering, we can surrender to a power greater than ourselves—"We will comprehend the word serenity. We will know peace," Bill W. wrote in *The Big Book of Alcoholics Anonymous.*

In illness, I did not learn these lessons immediately or fully, nor would I have wanted to. Just as cancer has become part of my journey, so has the healing of my spirit.

All the lessons have not been learned, indeed, will never be learned. There are days when I am stalled on the journey, days that I don't know why I ever began. But the latter implies a conscious choice, then an announcement of the trip, a bon voyage party and a setting off.

It did not happen that way. Instead, there was simply a growing awareness that a force I couldn't name was carrying me forward, slowly and easily. That I was being treated for cancer was not an impediment, but was perhaps the impetus for moving through life much more attentively than I had before.

What I saw, what I heard, what I felt with my heart I trusted, tentatively at first, then more fully. It is only in looking back that I see the enormity of the instruction that was given to me, and realize that it can all be distilled into some lessons that are, on their face, quite simple.

Yes, I heard voices, and this is what they said:

• *No, you're not as strong as you once were. So what?* When debilitating disease strikes an otherwise healthy person, the change is immediate and often difficult to come to terms with. Even if you weren't climbing mountains before you became sick, you can easily convince yourself that you would've—"If only this hadn't happened, I would have scaled Mount Everest."

Maybe, and maybe not. Or maybe you will still. But that is not what is likely to happen in the throes of illness. What you get is a powerful reminder that whatever mastery you believed you had over your body was an illusion. With the reminder, you can learn about humility and acceptance and compassion for yourself, all of which will nurture you in a healing way.

There is great strength in acknowledging weakness and limitations, because it can keep you grounded in reality. While the reality of illness may not be where you would've chosen to be, it is there that you have the opportunity to look at a mountain, admire its beauty, and dream of its heights; you don't have to climb it. It is about slowing down and paying attention to what your body tells you. It is about being in tune with the universe at ground level.

After you have acknowledged the physical limits that illness has created, there must also be an acceptance that those limits may be part of your life for a long while, perhaps always. This doesn't mean that you will become an invalid, but it means that even if you do—or if you do just for a while—your spirit and humanity are sailing on even though the vessel is listing.

- *You don't have to do it perfectly.* There is no right and wrong way to be sick. Stay in touch with your heart (the metaphorical one, as well as the one susceptible to myocardial infarction), and trust its wisdom. There is no one among us who is an authority on being human—we simply are human. All we can do is the best we can.

- *It's OK to be scared.* Five years after cancer, I do not yearn for the old breast, the old life. If cancer was the price I had to pay to make the transition to a place of peace, I would do it again in a heartbeat.

But I'd still be scared. They don't call it life-*threatening* for nothing—and fear is a common reaction to a threat against one's life (unless you're The Terminator or Indiana Jones).

Some of the fear is about what comes after diagnosis—fear of decision making, of treatment, of disability, of losing control. Looking back, I know that it was legitimate fear, because for almost four years my day-to-day life was dictated by cancer treatment and its effects. The key, for me, was to keep the fear in a comfortable balance with hope. I could not, as some Eastern thinker once said, keep the fear from landing, but I could keep it from making a nest in my hair.

• *The dishes can wait.* Give yourself permission to take care of yourself. Don't say "Yes" when you want to say "No." And don't feel guilty about it. We're so programmed to do, rather than simply to be, that even with the demands of illness, we find ourselves trying to figure out how to accommodate work, family, and chores.

Instead, we need to listen to that healing voice that will lead us to nurture ourselves on both sensory and spiritual levels. A hot bath and getting in bed with clean socks on was pure pleasure for me—I still don't have any explanation for the socks, but they made me feel secure. The dishes might be piled in the sink, the dust bunnies might be multiplying in the corners of every room, but I had clean socks.

When you make the commitment to nurture yourself, rather than doing what others expect (or what you, in the past, would have expected of yourself), you are acting with compassion—compassion for yourself, sans guilt.

• *This is your life.* Where am I now? Five years after the end of my treatment, a significant marker in the oncology world, there were no visible signs of cancer. Still, every six months the doctors look and look and look. They hope they don't find any errant cells— and I hope they don't find any—but they also don't want to overlook any. There is always a risk.

Every morning and every night for five years, I took a tiny 10 mg tablet of a drug called Tamoxifen, a chemotherapy drug that's used to treat some breast cancers after more aggressive treatment is over.

My cancer cells had positive estrogen receptors, meaning that in the presence of that hormone, they would grow, although slowly. Tamoxifen creates a false menopause, with all the attendant symptoms—hot flashes and dry skin among them. But it gave me a better chance of living a life without cancer for whatever years there are to be.

And, strange as it might sound, it is the life that cancer gave me that I am grateful for. Yes, it is different. Yes, it is uncertain. But it is blissful—blissful in the way of *ananda,* an ancient Sanskrit concept that suggests that all of life and death, joy and sorrow, agony and ecstasy taken together produce total happiness in our lives.

All we have to do is show up.

Carol

Sterna Citron, daughter of the late Rabbi Eli Chaim Carlebach, tells the story of the oil merchant Rachamim. Having extended heartfelt hospitality to the Hasidic master Baal Shev Tom, the merchant Rachimim was granted the blessing of his choice. Already living in comfort, he had but one wish: a guaranteed place in the world to come. Hearing this, the Baal Shem Tov sighed deeply, replying at last, "Assemble a large shipment of wine and bring it to my home."

This was no small task, given that the Baal Shem Tov lived far from Rachamim. But the oil merchant complied, leading his caravan of carts and drivers through towns, villages, and forests. One night, as rain suddenly burst from the heavens, Rachamim hurried down the road to find shelter for his load. Settling the carts and drivers in a large, empty warehouse, he then returned to a nearby inn to pass the night. In the morning, he rose early to rejoin his caravan, but something was terribly wrong. The warehouse was empty. There was no sign of the wine, the wagons, or the drivers. He hurried back to the inn, but it, too, had disappeared. Spying a group of men talking by the roadside, he hurried over to them: "Have I lost my way? Where is the inn of this village?"

The men looked at him, amused. "There is no inn near here," they replied.

Rachamim took the news heavily, sinking to the ground. "What am I to do?" he cried. He was far from home and family, having lost everything. As he lay in the dust, a group of beggars happened by and invited him to join them. Rachamim assented, never once succumbing to bitterness about his great loss.

The band of beggars wandered from village to village, arriving after many months in the hometown of the Baal Shem Tov. Sensing Rachamim's arrival, the Baal Shem Tov sent for him, preparing for him at his table the seat of honor.

"Do you remember the last time we met?" the Baal Shem Tov asked him at last. "You asked me for a share in the world to come. You believed that all you needed was my blessing. But my blessing, alone, could not prepare you for that which you've asked."

The Baal Shem Tov explained to those who had gathered that Rachamim had impressed him with his heartfelt hospitality. But having a good heart alone is not enough to warrant a place in the world to come. If one has a pleasant life, goodness can come easily. But to have everything taken away and not become bitter, this is how one becomes worthy of the blessing that Rachamim desired. The Baal Shem Tov continued, "On Sunday, Rachamim's wagons, wine, and drivers will find their ways back to him."

Sure enough, just as the Baal Shem Tov promised, Rachamim's worldly goods were restored to him. But as happy as he was to have them back, they meant little compared to his greatest attainment: a heart that had shown itself strong enough to sing a song of love and hope regardless of whatever fate sent his way.

When I was diagnosed with breast cancer, undergoing the rigors of chemotherapy, I admired the faith of Rachamim. But Rachamim is a story with a happy ending. There were no such assurances of full restoration in my own life. Could my heart sing nevertheless?

Sometimes. But it could also rage and shiver, cry and burn. In the end, my cancer gave me permission to explore my true human potential—the broader range of emotions that are found only beyond the boundaries of ordinary definitions of success and failure. Not just the simple pleasures of happiness or peace, but the deeper waters of passion, yearning, bittersweet sadness, and even despair. Again and again, I was asked to follow my faith off the edge of the cliff with only the endless mystery of the infinite to catch me. Will it always?

Here's what I learned: If you are sure that everything will turn out just the way you hope, then you are still clinging to the edge. The order you can envision for your life is quite simply not the order of the divine. To be fully alive is to rise and fall on ever-changing tides of dread and awe. When you become certain, you fall. When you are cast out, you are found. Only when you become willing to embrace the whole range of human experiences do you find the connection to the divine.

This, then, is sacred space: the realm of the true mystic. This is not tamed order, delivering you physical recovery in reward for your obedience. But rather, creation out of chaos, the terror of plummeting through deep mystery, wrestling with your own embarrassing finitude. And then, impossibly, there are those rare, sublime moments when you experience the in-breaking of God. As mystic philosopher Charles Kingsley writes, "When I walk the fields, I am oppressed now and then with an innate feeling that everything I see has a meaning, if I could but understand it. And this feeling of being surrounded with truth which I cannot grasp amounts to indescribable awe sometimes."

You can not make these moments happen. You can, however, place yourself in environments in which you can allow yourself to become receptive to experiences where the in-breaking of God is more likely to occur.

Penuel Ridge is one such place for me. A retreat center outside of Nashville, Penuel Ridge is named for the place where Jacob wrestled on the banks of the Jabbok River for God's blessing. Toward the end of chemo, I joined the Penuel Ridge community for a quiet day—a once-a-month opportunity for silent prayer and meditation in beautiful surroundings. There are open fields, hilly ridges, a simple whitewashed chapel hand-made of haybales, and my favorite destination: a shady wooded path that meanders around a small lake. It had rained the night before, stirring to life the lake's many turtles and frogs, kicking concentric circles onto the swollen lake's surface.

As much as I anticipated my walk around the lake, I sat on a bench close to the path's beginning to collect my thoughts before embarking. Between the bench and the path, water poured over the concrete spillway, feeding the creek below. So, too, my emotions overflowed my heart. The much-anticipated approaching end of chemo brought the joyous promise of relief from the chemicals that had temporarily drained the life from my blood. But it was also a time of terror, for I would shortly have done everything I could within my power to free myself from cancer. How was I to go on, living my life over the edge? With this thought, I was suddenly ready to walk. Without hesitation, I marched across the spillway and onto my journey around the lake. In my mind the words of Isaiah 43 repeated themselves over and over again: "Now says the Lord—Fear not, for I have redeemed you; I have called you by name, you are mine. When you pass through the waters, I will be with you; and through the rivers, they shall not overwhelm you; when you walk through fire you shall not be burned, and the flame shall not consume you...."

The sound of the luncheon bell woke me from my litany of hope, and I found my way back to the retreat center to eat my favorite bag lunch of crackers and cheese in silence. But as I approached the main house, I heard the alternating sounds of distress and consolation. I passed over the front stoop, strewn with mud-covered sneakers and a wet pile of jeans and a T-shirt. Inside, the Penuel Ridge staff huddled around one of the retreat regulars, Lorraine. The last time I'd seen Lorraine, she'd been seated quietly on a bench not far from mine at the lake. Now she was wrapped in towels, crying.

"What happened?" I asked, adding my concern to the chorus. Lorraine looked straight at me with such a strange mix of emotions, it sent shivers up and down my spine. Then everybody looked at me.

"They warned me that with the rains, the spillway was too slippery to cross," Lorraine gulped. "But then, while I had settled on sitting on the bench, I saw you get up and march across it without a moment's hesitation. I thought they must be mistaken. So I strode across it, just like I'd seen you do."

"So what happened?"

"On my very first step, I lost my footing, sliding down the spillway over the waterfall into the creek."

"She could have seriously hurt herself," one of the woman in the circle of healers commented.

Then there was silence. Obviously, Lorraine was scratched, wet, and shaken up. But she was not seriously injured. No, the silence was not for Lorraine, but for me. At last, she asked, "How did you get across when none else could?"

I did not have an answer, for there was no thought, no plan, no artifice involved. Isaiah 43: "I have called you by name, you are mine." At that moment, I had a sense that I was part of a whole, far greater than my fears about the end of chemotherapy and the possible recurrence of cancer. I felt that there had been moments—and that there would be more—where I unself-consciously became unified with God. I remembered the Sh'ma, the watchword of the Jewish faith: *Hear O Israel, the Lord Our God, The Lord is One.* And I understand that union with God is not the means to an end, but the end itself. The truth is that we do not always know where we are headed. We are destined to live portions of our life over the edge in mystery. But it is possible to be in a free-fall within the heart of the divine.

When I saw Lorraine a month later, she rushed to embrace me.

"Thank you, Carol. What happened to me that day changed my life!"

She told me that for years, she'd hated her name. In fact, she'd come to Penuel Ridge that day hoping to find a new name that would help her to feel more like herself.

"When I got home that night, I stumbled across a book of baby names I'd bought some time ago. Believe it or not, I'd never looked up my own name in the book. I couldn't believe what I read: In my own cultural tradition, Lorraine means 'waterfall.' The fall I took was my baptism. I'm finally at peace with my name—and it turned out to be my own."

That we do not feel unity with God consistently is not a sign of personal failure. As I learned from studying the books of Rabbi Abraham Joshua Heschel while pursuing my doctorate in religion, to reside in a constant state of oneness with the divine is the hallmark of the saint. For the rest of us, we find ourselves in a constant state of wavering, first soaring and then descending. At the peak, we feel whole and connected. In the valley, we despair of ever raising our heads above the mud. Yet there exists always the possibility that the divine will seek us out, in whatever state we may find ourselves.

Moments of unity can happen to you regardless of your circumstances. Even if you do not live permanently in such a state, once you have experienced the in-breaking of the divine, your life can begin to pivot around this new, higher center. You know what is possible for you. It's not that you give up your everyday life, envisioning goals, carrying out plans, celebrating or mourning the things that happen to you. But the drama of your individual circumstances is now played out against an all-encompassing love and mystery.

There is something infinitely freeing about having to live your life with no guarantees of any particular rewards—other than the connection to divine love that is always possible, regardless of your circumstances. After that day at Penuel Ridge, I was freed from the expectation that it was within my power to self-consciously control my destiny. All I could do was my part. God would have to take me the rest of the way. Sometimes I would cross the spillway. Sometimes I would slide down it. I had to trust that whatever my destiny, God was with me always.

As I have reentered the mainstream of my life, the ramifications of what I learned as a result of my cancer continue to unfold. I know now what it's like to feel embraced by God. Out of the fullness of this memory, I am free to take my pain, my sadness, even the inevitability of death, and make something awesome of it. What I choose to do with my freedom is to give my life to God, who wants only for me to be fully Carol Matzkin Orsborn for the rest of my life.

❧

On his journey to enlightenment, a student came across a spiritual master on the road outside the village.

"Teacher, I am doing everything I can think of. I pray. I meditate. I live in peace and I try to do what is right and good. What else can I do?"

The old teacher stood up and held his hands toward heaven. His fingers became like lamps of fire and he said, "If you will, you can become all flame."

Susan

It is breakfast time at Nashville's answer to a California coffeehouse. A cute little place with spaced-out guys behind the counter, unfamiliar with the menu, not quite awake. I order my double skinny latte and spy the fruit salad in the display case.

"Do you have fruit salad?" I ask.

"We don't have fruit salad, we just have fruit," is the response.

I point to the bowl of fruit salad in glass display case.

"Oh, that's the fruit."

I order a bowl of it.

This reminds me once again of the lessons of cancer. The lessons are unique for each of us. It comes down to how we interpret, what we feel, what we see, what brings us joy, and what causes pain. My joy was in discovering compassionate hearts where I least expected them and the healing balm of supportive friends. My deepest pain was psychological. The yawn of the nurse who was supposed to be counseling me felt like a stab wound. The anguish of telling my children that their mother has cancer.

The landmarks and feelings are continually surprising, like the adventure of taking a new hiking trail. I already know where the trail goes. At the end of it is my death. Comfort turns out to be an illusion. The only comfort is contentment with what is known, and with the unpredictable. Acceptance of the joy and acknowledgment of the pain. Reaching for the knowledge of my daily practice, joy and pain are one. There is nothing except God.

In this view, there is no distinction between practical and spiritual actions. As Inayat Khan writes, "Spirituality is enjoying and appreciating all things; understanding and comprehending everything; using and utilizing everything to its best advantage; surmounting difficulties; solving problems; clearing clouds of confusion and depression. Spirituality is fearlessness, joyfulness, calmness, and peace." Here is a list of some practical things that I learned from my experience with cancer:

• *Seek out an academic medical center, preferably one approved by the National Cancer Institute.* It may be large, cold, and on the wrong side of town. You will probably have to deal with minions of medical students. However, this is where the best science is done, and the most current treatments are offered.

• *Find a competent doctor.* Check credentials. Also ask on the grapevine.

• *Develop a relationship with your doctor.* Ask questions. Listen to answers. Ask for explanations.

• *Get a second opinion.* If your doctor resists this step, get a different doctor.

• *Find your best style for working with the medical system.* You may be like me and want to do your own research. You may want to put the decisions into your doctor's hands. It will probably be a combination of the two.

• *There is no one right way to make the choices.* Do not be hard on yourself. The decisions are an impossible dilemma. Do your best.

• *Find your voice.* I did this by writing in my journals. My meditation helped also. It kept me in touch with a stillness that was untouched by the commotion of illness. This is the same place that my voice comes from.

• *Ask for what you need.* This is your time to ask and to receive. I got this advice from a close friend and mentor who has lymphoma. She said, "If you want lamb chops in the middle of the night, ask for them." This is especially hard for those like me, who are used to nurturing others. Our asking enables people to give to us. We can give our gratitude, and tell of what we learned.

In the beginning of this book, I wrote about the sacred practice of "No." There is another version of this practice. It is the practice of "Yes."

I sit in my meditation posture. I have been here for several minutes, sinking into my pillow, following my breath, attuning to the subtleties of the inner world. With my eyes closed, my head makes a gentle circle. In the earlier practice, I exhaled, like sweeping away the cobwebs of illusion. Now, as I draw an invisible circle from my left shoulder, through my solar plexus, past my right shoulder, looking up, I inhale. I breathe in everything, the seen world and the unseen, the fullness and the emptiness, the unity and the diversity. If the practice ended here, I might become a puffball and float away. Instead, I turn my head downward, toward that point in my solar plexus, that place where the body is centered, where martial artists focus to get their strength.

All the fullness, all the breath, is focused in that limited center of a body that is not immortal, thats will die. The vastness is centered in the limited. The eternal is centered in the ephemeral. It makes no sense. That is the path of the mystic. "Make God a reality and God will make you the truth," says Inayat Khan. The reality of God is not just sweetness and light. The reality of God is all that there is.

The practice has not ended. But this is as far as my will takes me. I wait. And slowly, a feeling arises from that depth where all has been focalized. The feeling is as if I have bowed down, as low as I can. I bow my head to the ground, and surrender. Then, my head rises, but this time it is not of my will. It is as if gentle hands lift me up into a new world, one that I have never seen before. Where is that world? It is right here. I think of the words of Revelation, "Behold, I make all things new." The situation is the same as it was when I began my meditation, a few minutes before. Then what has changed? Touching the truth means seeing with new eyes. Rumi says that our vision of this reality is covered, like rust on a mirror. Our work is to clear away the rust. Spiritual practice scours the mirror. So does cancer.

The practice is not yet over. The fourth part is being still and listening. Listening for what? Listening for the sound of God's presence. This presence does not appear as a figure or an object. It is totally dispersed. It is in the sound of the wind, the rustle of leaves, and the tone of voice in a person who speaks from the heart. We are so immersed in this presence that we forget to notice. That is why this foundational practice of the Sufis is called "remembrance. "

Wake up! And remember. That is the essence of the spiritual path. The rest, as they say in mathematics, is the derivation. Through chaos, impact, choices, community, and spirit, what is it that we learn? Our lives become expressions of the sacred practice of "Yes."

Karen

When I write about what I have learned through cancer, I do not mean knowledge I could have gained in a classroom, and I also do not mean ideas that I have memorized and can now recite. Some of the things I list as lessons I already "knew." I mean that I believed them, and that as far as I was concerned, they were facts. But before cancer, I did not *know* these things in my bones; they were not a part of who I was. Now they are.

- *I have learned about suffering.* Of course I had suffered before I had cancer. But cancer familiarized me with a new level of suffering, and opened my eyes to how pervasive it is and just exactly how dreadful it can be. It is this awareness of suffering that finally connected me to every single human being on this planet. If nothing else, we are brothers and sisters because we all suffer.

  I also learned that no matter how horrible suffering is, God is able to bring some good out of it. My suffering has led me to see my life in a new way, and has given me a deeper enjoyment of and appreciation for each passing hour. This is true for more than just the suffering of serious illness. I have seen many people go through the suffering of divorce, for example, to exit on the other side happier, deeper people who know themselves much better. Even something so horrible as the Holocaust is not without some good. Of course the Zionist movement existed before World War II, but I think it was the Holocaust that brought world opinion to the state that enabled Israel to become established once again.

  Just as important, though, I have learned that with one exception, no new good thing created out of suffering is worth the cost of that suffering. I have heard some people say, "Gee, I'm glad I had cancer because I'm a better person now." I do not feel that way at all, not for myself, not for other cancer patients. Divorce may produce better people, but the pain is not worth the improvement. And even Israel is not worth the lives of six million Jews and the suffering of those who survived.

The exception I spoke of is the resurrection. It is a horrible thing to contemplate, but nevertheless I think it is a profound truth of the Christian faith: Somehow our suffering, combined with God's power, creates our resurrection. I suppose God could do things differently if she chose to, but this formula seems to have been true first for Jesus and then for everyone who has followed him.

• *I learned about loneliness.* It is not just losing friends that has made me feel lonely. I think illness necessarily creates loneliness. Flannery O'Connor said about her lupus, "In a sense sickness is a place, more instructive than a long trip to Europe, and it's always a place where there's no company, where nobody can follow."

The plain truth is that cancer makes me isolated. That is partly so because I was fairly young when I was diagnosed, but I doubt it would be much better if I were older. Cancer sets me apart from the vast majority of the people in my life ... all those who have never had cancer. Before I was diagnosed, my main concerns were similar to those of other people: work and love. I still have those concerns, but I have gained a new one, a concern that has a great deal of power. I am worried for my very life. Most people do not think about life and death every single day.

And the fact is that I am in a sense separated from even my closest, most faithful friends, from the people who are most able to have empathy for me. They can sit with me while I cry or worry, but when it comes right down to it, I was the one who had to get the treatments; I was the one who had to have the surgery; I am the one who will have to die from the disease.

I imagine my life these days as a long train trip through a featureless desert. There is no one else on the train with me, because no one else is traveling to the same destination I am. Every once in a while, I come across an oasis, and there the train stops for a bit and I spend time with someone I care about. Sooner or later, though, I have to hop back on the train and wave good-bye. I value those oasis times, but I have come to value the train time, too. I think all of us are riding on our own trains, like it or not. When life is "normal," we try to convince ourselves that our train is packed with family and friends, but I think it is more the case that normal life just means more oases. Sooner or later we all have to face the reality that we ride the train alone.

- *I learned that God is at the center of my life.* Since I am a minister, I have always been in the "God business." I have always taken the spiritual life very seriously. But cancer made me aware that God was at the very core of who I am and the days I live. I became aware that without that close and persistent presence, I would not even be able to breathe. It is God who sustains me.

- *I learned that the most profound faith looks the plainest.* Since I was a child, I have longed for a mountaintop experience of God: just one burning bush, just one little angel, just one experience that would let me know God was there. I read mystics' writings with passion while I was in seminary, and at one time I planned to focus my doctoral work on medieval women mystics.

The funny thing is that it is only since I have had cancer have I had any sort of experience that might be classified as mystical. This has happened twice. The first was after my first chemotherapy treatment. My fiancé drove me home and tucked me into bed. I had an incredible feeling of euphoria as I snuggled under the covers. I assumed this feeling was the result of some drug they had given me before the chemo itself, and I waited for it after each subsequent treatment. But it never came again. It had to be God; I cannot think of what else it might have been. The only grand message I took away from that encounter was "Everything is going to be all right." That message did not even come in words; it was simply a feeling. But things *were* all right, given the circumstances. I got through that first chemo and managed to gather the courage to go for the next one.

The second time I had a mystical experience was the day I went for my first two-month follow-up oncologist's visit. The doctor told me I had metastases in my lungs, and I knew I was going to die. I literally shook in terror while he examined me and wrote out a prescription for a tranquilizer. He went out to arrange a CT scan the next morning, and when he came back and led me out of the exam room, I suddenly had a wonderful feeling of peace pour into the top of my head and fill my body right down to my toes. Again, there were no words, just a feeling: "Everything is going to be all right." I felt this so strongly that I wanted to put my hand on my distressed doctor's arm and say, "Don't worry. It's not going to get me." These days, I know that it is true that "Everything is going to be all right," but that it does not necessarily mean my cancer will go away. For me to die and go to heaven is one possible way in which everything will be all right.

So I finally got my mystical experiences, minor league though they were. What I discovered, though, was that while they were important at the time, I have not centered my relationship with God on them. For one thing, trained as I am in psychology, I must necessarily question them. Were they from God, or did my distressed psyche manufacture some comforting experience?

But I also discovered that these experiences were relatively unimportant. If I had them all the time, I would have absolutely no trouble at all following God every moment of my life; I would have no anxiety about death; I would have all my questions answered—or perhaps I should say the questions would not matter anymore. In other words, I would have no need for faith. Clearly that is not the case for everyone, because there are some mystics who had and have those experiences for years. But not me.

I have also discovered another kind of spirituality; it is not of the mountaintop, but of the desert. This is a spirituality of endurance and nothing more. When it seemed that everything that could go wrong did, when I felt God had abandoned me, when there was little joy in my life, I still found myself believing in God. This was a God I was angry at— furious, I would even say. But my very anger necessarily meant I believed someone was there to receive the anger. My spirituality in the desert was simply an act of volition: "God, as far as I can see in my life, there is absolutely no evidence that you even exist. Nevertheless, I believe in you, and I believe you have good things in mind for me."

That prayer, said in the midst of a desperate feeling of abandonment, is the most profound spirituality I have ever experienced. It does not *feel* good in the way a mystical experience does, but it is rock-solid and indisputable. There is no turning back from it. I have come to the point that belief in and relationship to God is no longer an option for me; I am with God because that is who I am. There is no ecstasy in this kind of spirituality. But to endure in my world is a victory, a spiritual victory.

• *I learned that my value as a person has nothing to do with my accomplishments.* It is a long, complicated, and boring story, but I grew up believing that I was worth something because I was good at what I did—whatever I did. I was good at school, I was good at work, I was good at ministry, I was good at sex. Then cancer came along, and I was not good at anything any more. I could not work, I needed to receive compassion and care instead of giving it, my dissertation was not as good as it would have been if I had been well when I wrote it, and as for sex—well, who wants to sleep with a hairless woman with one and a half breasts? Yet there I was; here I am. God has preserved me, has sustained me, even though and even when I could not be good at anything. Apparently God cares about me even when I am a "loser."

I also learned that while God does, indeed, have a plan for my life, my worth does not depend on making progress on that plan. I still believe that God is personally, intimately involved in my life, as she is with every other person's, and has the best and wisest knowledge of what I am to do with my life in order to be happy and to help others. But even when it was impossible to figure out what that plan might be (Why am I still here?) and even when I could make no "progress," apparently God still cared about me.

I learned that at the most foundational level God loves me and I am a worthy person simply because I *am,* and because God chooses to regard me with love. I have learned that I cannot do anything—even fail—to change God's love for me.

• *I have learned the deep importance of reconciliation.* One of the side effects of being an Army brat and getting three degrees at different schools is that most of my friends are scattered across the country. I kept in touch with them during my treatment by sending out a cancer version of photocopied Christmas letters.

I wrote personal letters, though, to all the people with whom I had a ruptured relationship. If they had hurt me, I forgave them. If I had hurt them, I apologized profusely. If it was not clear what had happened to the relationship, I took all the blame. When I was staring death in the face, the issue of who was at fault became ridiculous.

I had good results with most of these letters. It was a huge relief to know that even if I were not going to have a continuing relationship with someone, we were able to end it on a positive and affectionate note. I had not realized before how much weight I had been carrying from broken relationships.

As with all these lessons, I still have not gotten this one down perfectly. There are two people I have not yet reconciled with, and that is because I am still angry with them. Right now, I have the luxury of believing that time will work some of that anger out, but there are never any guarantees on time, and I know it would serve *me* well to forgive these men and move on.

These lessons are only a few that I have taken from my life with cancer. There are perhaps a hundred more. I know the lessons will continue to come. I will soon be five years out from my diagnosis, and I still continue to learn.

Afterword

Carol

Throughout the spring and summer and into the early fall of 1998, the four of us grappled on our own with our answers to the challenging questions we had posed as a group. At last, the moment arrived when the task was complete and we were each able to read what the others had to say for the first time. Our agent handed the manuscripts around the table, along with neatly stapled piles of paperwork and sundry housekeeping tasks.

Coming as it did at the end of our busy workdays, despite the delicious chocolate chip cookies and fresh coffee, we were all in various states of exhaustion. In fact, I don't remember whether anybody stopped to celebrate the moment. Certainly, there were no toasts. If anything, I arrived at this momentous occasion feeling emptied out. Perhaps I was worried what the others might think about what I wrote.

And so it was that I returned home that evening, unopened manuscript in hand. While bed was calling out to me, I sat down in the big blue chair in my living room and decided to take just a little peek. To make a long story short, I could not put the manuscript down. Into the wee hours of the night I read, alternately laughing and crying. I forgot that reading through this first draft was "my job." Rather, the part of me that is still healing from breast cancer (and may always be) encountered every word as a balm to my sometimes lonely journey through serious illness. For here were three other women who understood the depths of what I had experienced. Not only that, but representing different stages of the illness, life experiences, and spiritual backgrounds, they answered many of the questions I had not even allowed myself to formulate. As I read, I felt alternately inspired and humbled. This was the book I had searched for in vain when I was diagnosed with breast cancer! And now, my vision had become a reality. I'm proud of the role I played in this. Of all the books I have birthed, midwifing this project is, I believe, my greatest accomplishment. I had known in my heart that these were three women whose voices had to be heard. My heart was right on.

In the end, I searched for the words that could best describe my response to the honesty and strength these three special women had shared with me, not only through their writing, but through the way they lived their lives. Nothing I came up with seemed adequate. And then, happily, an outside event intervened. Mark McGuire hit his sixty-first home run. I happened to catch him in an interview with a sports-caster. Mark was flushed with the joy of his accomplishment. Astonished at his own success, he finally grasped the words to convey his emotion. There was no embarrassment, no false humility, no holding back. "Wow! What a feat!" he cried out. He recognized the magnificence of his accomplishment and he allowed himself the well-deserved privilege of standing in awe before it.

Our accomplishment has nothing to do with sports. Nobody is going to get a million dollars for the ball we lofted over the wall. But you know what? *Wow! What a feat!* We have looked death straight in the eye and we have lived to tell our tales. Somehow, I believe the Earth has shifted just a bit on its axis because of us and that it is possible that the experience of serious illness will be forever changed for many people because of this book.

What have I learned from having breast cancer? I have learned that while it is true that unexpected bad things can happen to good people, it is also true that unexpected good things happen, too! For me, this book has been one of those good things.

Susan

When, at Carol's invitation, we met each other in the spring of 1998, I thought, "Finally, here is a real support group." We shared an approach to cancer that I had not found elsewhere. I had given up hope that there were kindred spirits on this path, initiates instead of warriors. In the space of an hour we were raucous and sober, giddy and sad, and committed to writing a book.

We agreed to write a sample chapter together. After that initial chapter, we would answer each question on our own. We met only a few times during the summer, to arrange logistics and navigate the technology adventures of word processors, faxes, and e-mail. It was always good to be together, to share the fear that comes with inconclusive diagnostic tests or inexplicable pain, to celebrate our project and our lives, and to eat chocolate chip cookies. We jokingly called ourselves the "Splice Girls," a reference to the surgical part of breast cancer treatment.

When I got my copy of the completed manuscript, I had the instinct to protect it. I felt that I held something holy. I took it home, and began to read, question by question. Alongside the other responses, I hardly recognized which parts were my own. I could not put it down. Carol's fight with Dan, Linda's friends in the room with her before surgery, Karen's shower after her Taxol infusion, my signing of the informed consent. These rich, honest details of illness were not recounted as laments, though as I read them, I cried. They were the ground of spiritual realization.

We wanted to call this book *How to Have Cancer Without Going to War,* to suggest a new language for the journey through life-threatening illness, a language of spirit instead of battle. In our stories, we tell of integrating the beauty of spiritual practice with the trials of cancer diagnosis and treatment. This is not automatic. Having a spiritual orientation or belief system is not enough. We know people dying from cancer who are entangled in a spiritual crisis, wondering what they did wrong or why God punished them. We hope our book can point a way through this anguish to a spiritual wholeness in illness as well as in health.

We pray for the day when cancer is eradicated, but until that time there will be more cancer initiates. We have much to learn from each other.

Now that you have heard our voices, what will you call us? What do we call ourselves? What language will we use? Are we victims? No way. Are we survivors? Perhaps, but that hardly describes the fullness of our experience. Are we thrivers? Too corny. Are we initiates? Yes, but this sounds a bit otherworldly, hardly a good introduction for the Kiwanis or the local high school. What will we say? To speak of cancer, we need a language for body and spirit. Introduce us as the ones who say, "Come what may."

Linda

There was fear after I had made the decision to share the story of my cancer diagnosis and treatment with three other women who had experienced those same life-changing words: *This is cancer.*

I had no concerns about how they would judge me, knowing absolutely that they would not. And, after all, I had already shared the story in another form in the newspaper I work for, a newspaper that went into almost 300,000 homes one Sunday morning on National Cancer Survivors Day.

But I did not then, and do not now, think of myself as a survivor. Nor a victim. Nor a sufferer.

I am a woman who is on a shared journey, and as I wrote about that path, knowing that my fellow travelers—Carol, Karen, and Susan— were with me, I began to realize that there is no right or wrong way to do it.

That had been my fear—that I had not learned enough, that I had not used the "opportunity" of cancer to grow. At the end of months of writing, however, I realized that we had all grown. There was no way to avoid it, should we have been inclined to. And we were all continuing to grow and change, to stop at various points along the way to comfort and to be comforted, to love each other and to love ourselves, drawing from a well that, in some bizarre way that is so often the case in nature, had been filled to overflowing from the shared experience of cancer.

By opening our hearts, in their wholeness and their woundedness, to each other, we received more of the abundance that we have been given, even as our lives as we have known them have been changed forever.

Karen

I am a very organized person—maybe neurotically so. I had plans for how to work on this book after we had all met on a Tuesday night and received our copies of the complete manuscript. I had cleared my Saturday and would read it then. On Monday, my day off, I would do whatever additional work was needed and take the manuscript to Linda Roghaar's house.

But here's what happened. I got home Tuesday night and started reading. I fell asleep on the manuscript—my drool marks prove it. I woke the next morning, immediately started reading again, and didn't stop until I was finished. Today is Friday, and I haven't been able to even think about writing my reaction until today. I was, for days, left absolutely wordless after my first encounter with the three-quarters of this book I had not written. I was and am overwhelmed by the strength, grace, depth, and wisdom of my coauthors. I wish I had known them when I was going through treatment. I envy you, the reader, because you *will* have that opportunity, even if you know them only by what they have written.

When I think of what I have read, what comes to my mind is not words but a picture. There is a tribe of remarkable women scattered all over the world. If I used the old battle language for cancer, I could easily call them Amazons—one-breasted warrior women—because the word *a-mazon* literally means "without breast." But instead what I see is a tribe of priestesses, each carrying around her a halo of shining wisdom. These women's beauty and radiance belie the pain of the initiation they endured: they were torn to the heart, physically, emotionally, and spiritually. The amazing light they bring has its source in those wounds. Their vocation as priestesses is to share their wisdom and their presence with those who are at the beginning of their initiations. This tribe of priestesses is not limited to my coauthors. It seems very unlikely that the only three women who have this quality should happen to live in Nashville and chance upon the same writing project. I imagine there are many more priestesses out there. I imagine one of them will be you.

Resources

Books

Albom, Mitch. *Tuesdays with Morrie: An Old Man, a Young Man, and Life's Greatest Lesson.* New York: Doubleday, 1997. A record of the author's weekly visits with his former professor, who is dying of Lou Gehrig's disease. Despite the fact that Morrie dies, this is an uplifting book that contains much of the same wisdom anyone with a serious disease comes to understand.

Dosick, Wayne. *When Life Hurts: A Book of Hope.* San Francisco: HarperSanFrancisco, 1998. Rabbi Dosick speaks from the richness of the Jewish tradition to provide comfort while exploring the mystery of God's presence.

Graham, Jory. *In the Company of Others: Understanding the Human Needs of Cancer Patients.* San Diego: Harvest/HBJ, 1982. Only for those with a terminal diagnosis! Graham speaks plainly about many of the fears, trials, and issues of those who have cancer. A hopeful, helpful book for those who feel they are alone or are "losing" to cancer. A bit dated on matters such as access to medical records, but at core, enduring.

Heschel, Abraham Joshua. *A Passion for Truth.* New York: Farrar, Straus and Giroux, 1973. Anything by Heschel will be of use to anyone who would like a serious engagement with Jewish theology. This book is a refreshing antidote to New Age superficialities, showing us that an honest and deep engagement with the God of the Jews includes struggle and sacrifice as well as joy.

Hirshfield, Jane, ed. *Women in Praise of the Sacred.* New York: HarperCollins, 1994. While much is said about patriarchy in the church, *Women in Praise of the Sacred* looks back at forty-three centuries of spiritual poetry by women. The work, from both Eastern and Western cultures, is not only eloquent, but also strong and hopeful.

Kaufman, Stuart. *At Home in the Universe: The Search for Laws of Self-Organization and Complexity.* Oxford: Oxford University Press, 1996.

Khan, Inayat. *The Complete Sayings.* Lebanon, NY: Sufi Order Publications, 1978. When experiencing the intensity of breast cancer, concentration is almost impossible. At the hardest times, poetry can be extremely helpful to calm the soul. From this book of short sayings comes a poem about joy arising at the end of sorrow.

Khan, Inayat. *The Path of Initiation* (Sufi Message of Hazrat Inayat Khan Ser: Vol. 10). London: Camelot Press, 1964. Note: out of print.

Kornfield, Jack. *A Path with Heart: A Guide through the Perils and Promises of Spiritual Life.* New York: Bantam, 1993. While one embarks on a spiritual journey with trust, Kornfield, like Hansel and Gretel, provides a trail for you—treasures that you will discover as you move toward integrating an increasing spiritual practice with your daily life.

Lewis, C. S. *The Chronicles of Narnia: The Lion, the Witch and the Wardrobe; Prince Caspian; The Voyage of the Dawn Treader; The Silver Chair; The Horse and His Boy; The Magician's Nephew; The Last Battle.* New York: HarperCollins Juvenile, 1994. This six-volume set of "children's" books is one of the best fictional explanations of the basics of Christian faith. Pays much attention to the problems of suffering. More hopeful and convincing than any sermon.

Lewis, C. S. *The Problem of Pain.* New York: Touchstone, 1996. A short, accessible Christian theological treatment of pain and suffering.

Love, Susan and Lindsey, Karen. *Dr. Susan Love's Breast Book.* Reading, MA: Addison-Wesley, 1995. Dr. Susan Love will surely bring out updated editions of this bestseller. Some of her advice and opinions are questionable. However, this book uses simple language to give a thorough description of medical breast cancer treatment complete with diagrams. Do not use this book for self-diagnosis, but as a reference only after you have met with a pathologist.

Markova, Dawnna. *No Enemies Within: A Creative Process for Discovering What's Right about What's Wrong.* Berkeley, CA: Conari, 1994. Presents a simple yet profound process for turning your problems into solutions, heartbreaks into breakthroughs, and internal enemies into allies.

Northrup, Christiane. *Women's Bodies, Women's Wisdom: Creating Physical and Emotional Health and Healing.* New York: Bantam, 1994. Dr. Northrup offers a medical perspective on every area of women's health, from problems to outcome. What sets this book apart, however, is that as she explains treatment options, she offers examples from her own work and life to show how a woman's spiritual and emotional state can affect treatment.

Nuland, Sherman. *How We Die: Reflections on Life's Final Chapter.* New York: Vintage, 1995.

Nuland, Sherman. *How We Live.* New York: Vintage, 1998.

O'Connor, Flannery. *The Habit of Being.* New York: Farrar, Straus and Giroux, 1979. The fiction writer's correspondence to friends about her work, her faith, and her eventually terminal disease, lupus. Hilarious in some places, extremely profound in others.

Oliver, Mary. *New and Collected Poems.* Boston: Beacon, 1992. Mary Oliver's poems are exquisite. This is the perfect book to keep nearby at all times. It evokes the particulars of life in the world that can feel so remote in the midst of a serious illness.

Orsborn, Carol. *The Art of Resilience: 100 Paths to Wisdom and Strength in an Uncertain World.* New York: Three Rivers Press, 1997. This is the book Carol Matzkin Orsborn was in the process of editing when she was diagnosed with breast cancer. The book consists of 100 readings from various religious and spiritual traditions that proved helpful to her and her readers in times of trouble.

Orsborn, Carol. *Solved by Sunset: The Right-Brain Way to Resolve Whatever's Bothering You in One Day or Less.* New York: Crown, 1996. A practical, self-guided retreat helping the reader to tap into her intuition to make decisions and resolve problems. Written by one of the authors of *Speak the Language of Healing,* this book is very useful for individuals who must make big decisions about treatment and deal with related issues in a deep and wise way.

Remen, Rachel Naomi. *Kitchen Table Wisdom: Stories That Heal.* New York: Riverhead Books, 1994. Remen speaks to doctors as well as patients. As a physician herself who suffers from serious illness, she shows by example how science and spirit can go together.

Rilke, Rainer Maria. *Selected Poems.* Trans. Robert Bly. New York: Perennial Library, 1981. Rilke has an amazing ability to get to the universal with very few words. His poetry helps one to maintain contact with the spiritual as it appears in the world.

Rinpoche, Sogyal. *The Tibetan Book of Living and Dying.* New York: HarperCollins, 1991. In Rinpoche's Buddhist practice, death is not something to be feared but something to be prepared for. This book gives precise descriptions of the states of consciousness of dying. Rinpoche gives instructions for *powa,* the breath practice for the moment of death. There is something comforting about approaching death in a practical instead of a mystical way.

Roberts, Elizabeth, and Elias Amidon, eds. *Earth Prayers from Around the World.* San Francisco: HarperSanFrancisco, 1991. Open this book and pick a prayer to say.

Rumi, Jelaludin. *Essential Rumi.* New York: HarperCollins, 1997. Rumi teaches us how to ask the right questions. His ecstatic poetry is a connection to the everlasting spirit of life.

Rumi. *The Illuminated Rumi.* New York: Broadway Books, 1997. These Rumi poems are set as jewels. This is a good book to hold on to, even without reading it.

Siegel, Bernie. *How to Live between Office Visits: A Guide to Life, Love and Health.* New York: HarperCollins, 1993. No matter how serious your prognosis, this book is full of stories of people who have learned to live every minute of life with meaning, humor, and love.

Speigel, David. *Living beyond Limits: A Scientific Mind/Body Approach to Facing Life Threatening Illness.* New York: Times Books, 1993. David Speigel is one of the leading psychiatrists in breast cancer support. His book is written with a feeling for those who will be reading it for support. It is filled with stories about how people approached their illnesses in spiritual ways.

Music and Audiotapes

Brown, James. "Get Up Offa That Thing, Dance and You'll Feel Better."

Chapman, Beth Nielsen. *Sand and Water.* Chapman wrote the pieces on this CD after her husband died of cancer. Obviously, they are from the perspective of the one left behind rather than the one with cancer, but the songs can help you grieve the many losses involved with cancer.

Hoffman, Janalea. *Musical Acupuncture.* An innovative concept in music therapy. Experience how music can conduct and move energy in your body in a way that's very similar to an acupuncture treatment without needles. This cassette has proven to be particularly effective for chronic pain such as arthritis, back pain, or headaches. *Side 1:* An interesting experience even for those who have trouble imaging. *Side 2:* All music. Instruments used: cello, flute, harp, bells, violin, and alto recorder. To order, see Rhythmic Medicine, under other resources, below.

Part, Arvo. *De Profundis.*

Part, Arvo. *Tabula Rasa.*

Stratos. A wonderful group of classical musicians who play without a conductor. Their CD contains music from the joyful and uplifting to the sad and sorrowful.

Sweet Honey on the Rock, 20th Anniversary, "Can't Know One Know."

Zuleikha, *White Pavilion.*

Online

Please note: We have not included URLs because they change so frequently. You should be able to find these sites with any search engine.

Breast Cancer ListServer

> This is an open discussion list for any issue relating to breast cancer. An unmoderated list open to researchers, physicians, patients, families, and friends of patients, for the discussion of any issue relating to breast cancer. WARNING: The list can generate 50–150 messages per day. Send e-mail to: LISTSERV@morgan.ucs.mun.ca—in the body of the message, type SUBSCRIBE BREAST-CANCER followed by your real name. For example, SUBSCRIBE BREAST-CANCER Jane Q. User.

Grateful Med

National Breast Cancer Coalition

National Cancer Institute

Oncolink—University of Pennsylvania

Other Resources

Gilda's Club

> A free emotional and social support community for men, women, and children with any type of cancer, their families, and friends. Named for Gilda Radner. Clubs in many cities. Contact the headquarters: Gilda's Club NYC, 195 West Houston, New York, NY 10014.

National Center for Jewish Healing

> 9 East 69th Street, New York, NY 10021. Phone: (212) 535-5900.

Rhythmic Medicine

> Since Janalea Hoffman founded Rhythmic Medicine in 1978, the organization's goal has been to raise awareness among the general public of specific ways music can be used therapeutically, as a natural alternative for emotional and physical health care challenges. Address: 11445 Craig, Overland Park, KS 66210.

Group Study Guide

S PEAK THE LANGUAGE OF HEALING lends itself to either individual or group study. The following exercises and discussion questions are designed to help small groups or classes work through the subject matter of this book, one session at a time. Individuals may also find value by studying these questions and adapting the exercises for personal use. While this study guide was written for people who have serious illnesses, the questions and exercises can easily be adapted for family members and friends or for individuals and groups who have a more general interest in the subject matter.

Many groups like to meet once a week for ten weeks, and consider one section of this study guide each week. One hour a week is sufficient, but each week's material could easily expand to fill two or three hours or even more. Feel free to experiment with one- or two-day retreats, ten consecutive evenings, or any other format that suits your needs.

In the suggested ten-session format, you may wish to ask group members to read the introductory material prior to the first gathering. During the subsequent nine sessions, you will work through each of the nine sections in turn.

Depending on the length of each session and the interest of the group, you may want to spend more time on some questions and exercises and less on others. Individual questions were written to reflect a variety of religious and spiritual orientations. Feel free to select and adapt the suggestions to your own group's needs and desires.

WEEK 1: INTRODUCTION

Discussion Questions

1. Have you encountered books or literature about cancer or other illnesses that use warfare terminology? What were they called? How did you respond? Were you inspired? Turned off?

2. The Greeks had a myth about a group of one-breasted warrior women called the Amazons. Does knowing this make war language more helpful to you? Or do you still prefer the image of cancer as initiation? If you don't like either, what image works for you?

Exercises

1. Get some paper, crayons, or pencils, and draw your experience with cancer. Don't start with a preformed image—and don't worry about the quality of the artwork. Just draw what the experience has felt like to you. Time permitting, do several versions of your drawing, and see whether an overarching image of your experience emerges from your art. (With this and many of the exercises to follow, you may want to play calming instrumental music in the background. Works by Vivaldi are a good choice from the classical music world. New Age music, particularly piano soloists, also works well.)

2. Design the ideal invitation to an illness-related fund-raiser that doesn't use warfare terminology.

WEEK 2: DID I CREATE THIS?

Discussion Questions

1. Are you holding any "if only's" in your mind about the cause of your illness? Such as, "If only I had been a vegetarian, if only I meditated every day, if only I lost weight." What are the grounds for these assumptions, if any? What would it be like if you let go of these "if only's"?

2. What unproven theories have other people come up with to explain how you created your illness? Did these theories help you or hurt you?

3. Do you believe that God is all-good and all-powerful? Or is your thinking similar to the ideas of process theology, which suggests that God doesn't stop evil in the world because God cannot: that God is not all-powerful in the way we've traditionally thought? (This is the point of view Rabbi Harold Kushner takes in *When Bad Things Happen to Good People.*) Or are you somewhere in between? On what do you base your beliefs about God's goodness and power?

Exercises

1. Choose a partner. Each partner takes a turn telling the other what he or she is going through. In each case, the listening partner remains attentive but silent, resisting the urge to solve the problem or provide a theory. After each partner has had the opportunity to both share and listen, discuss how it felt to be listened to without interruption. Was it harder to share or harder to resist offering advice or explanation?

2. Get a small ball of modeling clay, preferably clay you can bake and preserve. Relax as much as possible, and allow the thoughts that try to take hold of you pass through your mind. When you feel relaxed, turn your thoughts to God. While you are doing this, keeping your eyes closed, let your fingers shape the clay. When you're finished, open your eyes and see what you have created. Keep your piece as a visual reminder of this experience and to remind you that you are not responsible for your illness.

3. *The Practice of No.* In Susan's response to this question in the book, she talks about "The Practice of No." If you would like to try out this ancient mystical meditation for yourself, begin by siting quietly in a chair or in a meditative posture on the floor. Be attentive to your body. With each in-breath, notice your physical state, then your emotions. With each out-breath, gently release with a soft out-breath or sigh. Once you are quiet, move

your head gently in a circle, starting from the left shoulder, through the heart, to the right shoulder, and then upright. As you move your head, gently think "No," about the assumptions with which you view the world. Feel as if you are sweeping away cobwebs from your mind. Have the feeling that you are participating fully in the events of your life, but that you are more than just these events. There is nothing more you need to do. Clearing away these cobwebs allows you to see with fresh eyes. Repeat at least several times. (More, if possible.)

WEEK 3: DOES DEATH MEAN I LOSE?

Discussion Questions

1. What would it mean to you to be healed? Is being healed the same as being cured? Are there other ways of being healed besides on the physical level?

2. Have you found that some people in your life are frightened by you as a sick person? Why do you think that is? When you have known people who were seriously ill, what have your reactions been? Can you think of some way to be less frightened by mortality?

3. What do you think happens to us after we die? What does your spiritual or religious tradition (if any) teach? Do you agree? If you don't know or don't agree, is there some place or somebody you can turn to for guidance?

Exercises

1. Think of someone you know who is seriously ill, and think of how you can respond to her or him the way you wish someone had responded to you: send a card, make a phone call, listen without interrupting, give her a present. If you have materials on hand and are so inspired, make something that you then deliver in person.

2. Describe someone you know personally, or someone you have read about or seen in the media, who has faced a big challenge

in her or his life with a style you admire. (If you can plan in advance, have everyone bring in a picture, special object, or written material that says something about the person.)

3. Are you confused or conflicted about mortality? Perhaps you have an interior "board of directors" who have varying points of view. Listen to the voices in your interior dialogue as they discuss feelings and thoughts about dying. Do you have a Sufferer? A Mystic? A Scared Child? A Martyr? Is there a voice representing anger? Bewilderment? Can you hear your voice of Wisdom? Is there a voice of Peace? You can write down a dialogue between the voices in the form of a play. Or you can select various people in your group who remind you of your inner voices and ask them to play a part in an improvisation. (Wisdom and Peace get the final word!)

WEEK 4: DOES GOD GET TO VOTE?

Discussion Questions

1. When it comes to approaching challenges, do you get proactively involved, or do you prefer to let the chips fall as they may? Do you think one approach is better than the other, or does it make sense to find balance between the two?

2. Think about the issue of control in your life. Examine your feelings about independence and dependence. What does each of these mean to you? What values do you hold for each one; for example, is independence good and dependence bad? Can you see them related as interdependence?

3. Have you involved God in making decisions about your treatment and life? If you have, what methods have you used? Does knowing that you've tried to discern what God wants give you more peace about your decisions than you would otherwise have?

Exercises

1. Carol tells the story of the Zen master pouring tea for his disciple. He told the student that in order to receive, the student had

to first empty the cup. If you could empty your cup to make room to receive, what would you let go? Draw a picture that symbolizes something you would like to let go, and then share it with the group. At the conclusion of your meeting, think of some way to release the picture. (Burn it? Fold it into a paper airplane and sail it away?) If possible, go ahead and release it now as part of an improvised group ritual. If not, make plans to find a time and place to do so either individually or as a group.

2. Think of yourself right here and now, wherever you are. Come up with a list of the things that you are dependent upon: air, water, the beating of your heart, the food you've eaten today, and so on. After making this list, reconsider the broader concept of what it means to be dependent, independent, and interdependent.

3. Karen's reading suggestion: *The Spiritual Exercises* by Saint Ignatius of Loyola. Find and read to the group his brief passage called "Discernment of Spirits," wisdom for those who are trying to make a decision and feeling anxious about it. If you are in a retreat setting, follow this by a period of prayer, meditation, or walking in nature.

WEEK 5: IS TREATMENT WAR OR INITIATION?

Discussion Questions

1. Do you think that the goal of resilience is to emerge from life's experiences unchanged, or to be somehow transformed by them?

2. How has your illness changed you? Are the changes worth what you've been through? What have you had to sacrifice, and what have you gained?

3. Susan quotes Inayat Khan: "Sometimes initiation comes after great illness, pain or suffering. It comes as an opening up of the horizon and in a moment the world seems transformed. It is not that the world has changed, but the person is tuned to a different pitch. She begins to think, feel differently, and to act differ-

ently. Her whole condition begins to change. One might say, from that moment, this person begins to live." What does this quote mean to you? What do you think it means to say, "This person begins to live?" How do you know when you have had an initiation?

Exercises

1. Write a letter of gratitude to a part of your body that is experiencing challenges now (or has in the past), thanking it for the positive role it has played in your life.

2. If you were going to write a book about your life, what would the chapter titles be? Earmark those events that changed you forever. These might be major events such as marriage, divorce, death of a loved one; or they can be events that were insignificant on the surface, yet transformed you. See if you can come up with ten or more chapter headings to share with the group.

3. Homework: If possible, prior to this session, visit a library and take a look at Joseph Campbell's volumes on myths. The myths that resonate most strongly with the battle image for illness are what Campbell collects under the heading, "The Hero's Journey." Look beyond to his volume on mother goddess myths. Take the time to look through it, discovering the tales that catch your imagination and give you a new way to envision your illness. Make a copy of your favorite story (or take notes) to share with the group.

WEEK 6: DO I HOLD ON OR LET GO?

Discussion Questions

1. Do you have an easy or difficult time relying on other people and other sources of strength? Why do you think this is true for you?

2. Have you found yourself angry with or alienated from God since your illness? What did you learn about anger at God when you were growing up? Try to remember a specific source: a sermon, a religious school teacher, your parents? When you feel

angry with God, do you also feel guilty? How would it be if you could leave this guilt behind?

Exercises

1. Make a wish list of things you want and need. If you can't think of whom to ask to help you get what you need, ask the group to help you brainstorm ideas.

2. Skim the Psalms for ones where the author expresses anger or even rage. Share them out loud, with feeling, with the group. Try writing your own psalms and share these, as well.

WEEK 7: DO I TRUST THE MEDICAL ESTABLISHMENT OR SHOULD I PUT MY FAITH IN ALTERNATIVE AND SPIRITUAL HEALING?

Discussion Questions

1. What do you think "medical establishment" refers to? What do you think of as "alternative" or "spiritual healing" practices?

2. Do you or have you had a "magic bullet"—something you believed could guarantee that you get the result you want? What is the difference between superstition and hope?

3. Do you believe in miraculous healing? Why or why not? If you do, what do you think determines who gets healed? Is this fair? Do you feel free to be open with your family, friends, and faith community about your beliefs?

Exercises

1. Imagine the perfect healing environment, tailor-made just for you. What does it look like? What does it feel like? What does it smell like? Sound like? Who is there with you? What happens to you when you are in this place? Draw a picture or write a description of this place.

2. Choose a partner and discuss the answer to these two questions: In relation to the biggest challenge I am facing right now, what

can I change? In relation to the biggest challenge I am facing right now, what must I accept?

3. If you are in a retreat setting, bring in a masseuse (or give each other good shoulder massages). If you are working these questions and exercises through individually, treat yourself to a massage this week. Plan some quiet time after your massage. Let your mind wander, and pay attention to the way you feel. Are you having more feelings than you would have expected? Where did all these feelings come from?

WEEK 8: FROM WHOM MUST I LEARN
TO RECEIVE? FROM WHOM MUST I LEARN
TO PROTECT MYSELF?

Discussion Questions

1. When you were newly diagnosed with a major illness (or remember when you were first diagnosed), did you tell people? Why or why not? Whom did you find it easy to tell? Whom did you avoid?

2. Think about the people who have been involved in your life since the illness. Have you been either pleasantly or unpleasantly surprised by the ways some of them have reacted? What are the most helpful things people have said or done to or for you? What things troubled you, even if they were well intended?

3. What are some things you should *not* do when somebody you know is diagnosed with a serious illness?

Exercises

1. Find a partner and create a comic skit in which a visitor to a hospital room does as many things wrong as possible. Present the skits to the group. (How about serving popcorn?)

2. Think of the person who has made you the angriest since your illness. Who has been the most thoughtless, the least empathetic? Write that person an angry letter. Don't leave anything out. Use the worst language you know, and call him or her

every name you can think of. Then put the letter away. Notice how you are feeling now. Are you angry or sad? (Mark on your calendar to revisit this letter in a month. Now what are your feelings? Have they changed?)

3. Reread the story of Tikkun Olam in Susan's response to these questions (p. 145–6). How do you feel about this story? How is your world broken, and where is it being knitted together?

WEEK 9: HOW CAN I FIND PEACE OF MIND WHEN I'M LIVING MY LIFE OVER THE EDGE?

Discussion Questions

1. What does it mean to live your life over the edge? What does this have to do with the idea of initiation or awakening? Is there a difference between living your life over the edge and peace of mind? Can you have both of these simultaneously?

2. Why do you think, in some Eastern spiritual practices, people meditate in graveyards? What could the spiritual benefits be?

3. Do you accept the reality of your death? If so, what is that like for you? What feelings does it bring up? If you don't, what do you believe this denial gains you? If you are fearful about death, is there someone who will let you talk about it, not minimize your anxiety, but also be hopeful?

Exercises

1. If possible, use part of your time together to sit quietly in a sacred place. It could be indoors, in a library or sanctuary, or outdoors in nature. If it isn't possible to leave the group space, you might work to create a sacred environment by turning the lights low, playing inspirational music, and lighting candles and/or incense. People can close their eyes, or read randomly from *Speak the Language of Healing* (or any other book or text) silently. At the end of the silent period, individuals can share their experience of sitting silently with the group.

2. Write your own list of "essentials," the important things in your life that you cannot do without. (Take the list out periodically in the future and see if and how your list of "essentials" changes over time.)

3. Now, as we near the conclusion of this series, revisit your earlier thoughts about the metaphors commonly used in the world of serious illness. What other metaphors besides life as a battlefield could you now use to describe your experience? A garden? A painting? A story? A dance? Is there a place for the concept of death in these metaphors? (Remember Carol's colorful fish with purple eyes!) Write or draw a metaphor that works for you.

WEEK 10: WHAT HAVE I LEARNED?

Discussion Questions

1. What does it truly mean to fulfill your human potential? What qualities, experiences, and characteristics are you now willing to honor and include in your life that you once may have thought of as undesirable?

2. Has going through your illness changed your faith? On the continuum of sunny optimism versus gloomy pessimism, where would you put yourself now? (Do you have different names for the extremes of your own personal faith continuum?) Do external events move you up or down the continuum? Do you have in place spiritual practices or resources that you can call upon? If not, if you wish you did, where and how could you begin to develop them?

3. What does it mean to be on a "spiritual path"? Is there a difference between actions that you take to be "spiritual" and those you think of as not spiritual? How could illness as well as good health—accompanied by all the feelings and experiences that come with each—both be considered to be part of your spiritual path?

Exercises

1. Guided Meditation: Relax as much as possible, breathing slowly and deeply. If you feel comfortable, close your eyes. (The group leader reads this next portion out loud.) Now, imagine yourself in a peaceful, quiet library. How does the library smell? Are there windows, or are you in a dark, private space? Are there comfortable chairs? Tables? What is your favorite place in the library where you can curl up and read? Imagine the color of the chair. The fabric. The temperature in the room and the quality of the light. Now imagine: Where are the books? Are they all around you, or do you take an elevator up or down to get into your favorite stacks? Imagine yourself going to where the books are, wandering happily through the stacks looking for a special book. Suddenly, you recognize one that has your name printed on the spine. You take the book eagerly off the shelf, and bring it back to the most comfortable, inviting chair in the library. Now, open it. Keep your mind open as the book tells you what wisdom you have to share with others. Be prepared to be surprised. The wisdom may come as words on the page, or it may be a picture of an object, abstract shapes, or simply a feeling. You don't have to understand it for your book's contents to have value. When you are ready, open your eyes and journal about this experience. At the conclusion, share what you "read" with a partner, or with the group as a whole.

2. Plan some kind of celebration. Perhaps a potluck meal or dancing together to upbeat music. Invite people to bring or make a sacred object that symbolizes your spiritual journey to share with the group.

3. *The Sacred Practice of Yes.* Sit quietly. Close your eyes. Gently make a circle with your head from left to right while inhaling, feeling yourself becoming part of all things. When your head reaches the top of the circle, exhale softly while bowing your head. Feel as if you are embraced by a compassionate presence, like dissolving in the arms of a friend. Then raise your head slowly, so your closed eyes are pointed straight ahead, trying to

sense a subtle hint of something fresh and new, like the scent of grass at dawn. Breathe naturally. Feel a sense of sacred presence within you and around you. Realize that with every moment comes a fresh dispensation of life and possibility. This experience of divine presence, no matter what the outward circumstances of your life, is the sacred practice of Yes. Repeat at least several times, more if possible.

4. Write your list of "What have I learned?" Share it with the group, your family, friends, your physicians and nurses.

5. Discuss whether you'd like to continue meeting together in some way. What questions would you like to revisit? What issues have yet to be addressed? Would you like to meet periodically just to stay in touch? If you do want to continue, it's useful to plan a specific date to get together again before you officially end your studies.

For Further Study

For updated information on workshops, retreats, groups, and talks inspired by *Speak the Language of Healing,* or to contact the authors via e-mail, visit their web site at **www.speakhealing.com**. To arrange for an appearance by one or more of the authors, call Karen Stroup at (615) 255-9903 or e-mail stroupkl@aol.com.

If you or your group would like to continue your self-study, Carol Matzkin Orsborn's book *Solved by Sunset* is a self-guided workshop on the subject of intuitive decision making, designed for individuals or groups to work through together in a one- or two-day retreat setting. She has also written a group study guide for *The Art of Resilience* for use in a ten-session format. If you would like a free copy of the guide, send a SASE to Resilience, The Orsborn Company, P. O. Box 159061, Nashville, TN 37215.

Acknowledgments

OUR GRATITUDE GOES TO OUR AGENT LINDA ROGHAAR, who had the depth of wisdom and compassion to recognize the need for this book in the world. Her faith in what we came together to do was unflagging. Through her devotion to this project, she saw us through completion of the writing process and found us a great publishing partner: Conari Press.

We salute the vision of the staff at Conari for their enthusiastic support. We are proud to be in partnership with you.

SUSAN KUNER:

To Carol, Karen, and Linda for your courage, your honesty, your laughter, and the privilege of working together. To my husband, Vakil, my children, Afsal and Satya, my sister, Rae Grad, my brother, Dennis Krohn, my mother, Edith Krohn, my family, friends, and coworkers for gathering around and staying close. To physicians who grow in compassion as well as skill, especially my surgeon Dr. Daniel Beauchamp of Vanderbilt University Medical Center and my consulting physician, Dr. Alan Rabson of the National Cancer Institute. To Pir Vilayat Khan and my friends in the Sufi Order International who are joyously engaged in the spiritual laboratory called life.

CAROL MATZKIN ORSBORN:

To "Em," a composite character who appears throughout this book. In truth, Em includes the following wise women who midwifed my initiation into spiritual maturity: my friends and coauthors Susan Kuner, Karen Leigh Stroup, and Linda Quigley. My divinity school classmates, particularly Emily Askew and Tanya Marcovna. My spiritual advisors Marjorie Thompson, Mary Faulkner, and Joan Fuhrman.

To all those big-hearted Nashvillians who supported me and my family through treatment, including the Congregation Micah, Penuel Ridge, and the Vanderbilt University Divinity School communities. Special thanks to Wendy Kanter and Deborah White and to the parents of Jody's friends who filled in all the empty spaces. Gratitude, too, to Gilda's Club—a great new addition to Nashville's growing healing community.

To my crack medical team, including my California advisors: my brother Dr. Gene Matzkin, my father and mother Dr. Lloyd Matzkin and Mae Matzkin; and the compassionate pros at Vanderbilt University's medical facility; particularly, Dr. Daniel Beauchamp, Dr. David H. Johnson, Research Nurse Norma Campbell, Carol Caillouette and all the caring nurses at the chemotherapy treatment center. You shined a bright light into all the scary places. Thank you.

Finally, I thank my family—my husband, Dan, my son, Grant, and my daughter, Jody. Your love held me in God's embrace—and holds me still. We were all initiated by my cancer and I am humbled by the strength and brilliance of your faith in me, in yourselves, and in life.

LINDA QUIGLEY:
Even though I make my living with words, sometimes there are none that can say enough. What will have to do is to say thank you with all my heart to my parents, Gene and Lois Quigley; my brother, Brooks Quigley; my physicians, Drs. Bonnie Miller, Joe DeLozier, Patrick Murphy, and Paul Rosenblatt, and their staffs; therapists Lynn Hancock, Kittie Myatt, and Jennie Adams; my friends, old and new, my co-writers on this book, and my colleagues at the *Tennessean;* and to Mary Jones and Lois Green, who showed me the way then and are showing me still. And to Angela Smith, I give love and thanks abundantly and always.

KAREN LEIGH STROUP:

I have said in my writing that I would not be the person I am without the initiation of cancer. I also would not be who I am now without the contributions of many people. I would like to acknowledge them here: for keeping me alive, with great kindness and respect, the Vanderbilt Cancer Center, especially Dr. David H. Johnson and Patti Higgins, R.N.; for serving as my pastors during the worst of my disease, Dr. Liston O. Mills and Dr. Lanny C. Lawler; for collegial support and encouragement, Dr. Volney P. Gay; for hanging onto me while I dangled in the pit of suffering, my true, abiding friends, Heather Wibbels, Carol Sumner, Dave Krinsky, Tim Ellsworth, and Sharyn Dowd; for the comfort that only common experience can bring, the members of the St. Thomas Hospital cancer support group, those both living and dead; and for the invitation to join in this project and their continuing support, Susan Kuner, Carol Matzkin Orsborn, and Linda Quigley.

Index

About the Authors

Susan Kuner, Ed.D., is the Director of Vanderbilt University's Virtual School in Tennessee and is writing a book on patient care. The founder of Overachievers Anonymous and head of her own public relations firm in Nashville, Carol Matzkin Orsborn, M.T.S., is a well-known author whose books include *The Art of Resilience* and *Return from Exile*. Linda Quigley is a Pulitzer Prize-nominated journalist, also living in Nashville, who has won awards for a first-person account of her experience with breast cancer. Karen Leigh Stroup, M.Div., Ph.D., is the minister at Central Christian Church in Nashville, Tennessee, and a respected speaker on living with cancer.

Conari Press, established in 1987, publishes books on topics
ranging from psychology, spirituality, and women's history
to sexuality, parenting, and personal growth. Our main goal
is to publish quality books that will make a difference
in people's lives—both how we feel about ourselves
and how we relate to one another.

Our readers are our most important resource,
and we value your input, suggestions and ideas.
We'd love to hear from you!

To request our latest book catalog,
or to be added to our mailing list, please contact:

Conari Press
368 Congress Street, Fourth Floor
Boston, Massachusetts 02210
www.redwheelweiser.com

800-423-7087   fax 877-337-3309